# Snoring & Sleep Apnea

## Easy Ways To Stop Snoring

Frank Fletcher

## Warning and Disclaimer

Every effort has been made to make this digital book as complete and as accurate as possible, but no warranty or fitness is implied. The information provided is on an "as is" basis. The author and the publisher shall have neither liability nor responsibility to any person or entity with respect to any loss or damages arising from the information contained in this digital book.

The content of this digital book is based upon research conducted by the author and is being presented to you for educational purposes only. The content of this digital book is not intended to diagnose or prescribe for medical or psychological conditions nor to claim to prevent, treat, mitigate or cure such conditions.

No attempt is being made to provide diagnosis, care, treatment or rehabilitation of individuals, or apply medical, mental health or human development principles, to provide diagnosing, treating, operating or prescribing for any human disease, pain, injury, deformity or physical condition.
The information contained in this digital book is not

# Table Of Contents

# What Is Sleep Apnea?

For most, this is a term that is not well known. There are a number of different reasons that you may have found yourself learning about this condition. You may have been recently diagnosed or know of someone that has been. Or, you may be wondering if you are having these episodes yourself. The fact is that many suffer from it or may be having the early symptoms of it and they may not even realize it. Although that is the case for many, it doesn't have to be for you. Sleep apnea is a serious condition and should be taken with heart. But, before you become overwhelmed with your own needs, take the time to learn more about this condition so that you can improve your situation.

Sleep apnea is actually a disorder that happens when you are sleeping. You may have heard it called sleep apnea as well. In either case, the end result is the same. It is characterized by the fact that you have pauses in your breathing while you are sleeping. When this happens the episodes are called apneas.

This term actually means without breath. The seriousness of your condition is defined, at times, by how long these episodes actually last. For some, it is just one missed breath while for others it can be many more. The bottom line is that this happens many times while you are sleeping and that leads to all sorts of complications, as you can imagine.

There are actually two different types of sleep apnea that you may be experiencing. Central and Obstructive are the two differences. In Central, you will find that the problem is caused by a lack of effort by your body. With Obstructive sleep apnea, there is something that is blocking or obstructive your ability to breathe properly.

If you are experiencing problems with breathing and you think that you may have sleep apnea, there is help out there for you. The first thing to do is to educate yourself and then seek out the help of a skilled doctor in the field. Testing can easily be done to help you to determine if this is something that is happening to you. In either case, it is necessary for you to find the solution to this problem as it can worsen.

# Treatments For Central Sleep Apnea

If you have been diagnosed with central sleep apnea, then you already know just how serious your condition is. In this type of sleep apnea, your brain does not function as it should while you are asleep. It does not communicate with your muscles that they need to breath and that will cause you to wake up. When you do awake, you are likely to feel a shortness of breath. When this happens several times per night, it is important to talk to your doctor about the possible reasons behind it. If in fact central sleep apnea is the cause, then the doctor will work with you to find the right solution.

There are a number of different things that can be done to help improve your quality of life and minimize your risks of further problems. Although the treatment options for central sleep apnea are much less, they can work for those that need them.

- **_Medical problems treated._** Since many times this type of sleep apnea happens due to some other medical condition it is necessary for those to be improved in order for the sleep apnea to be reduces. If you have such things as heart or neuromuscular disorders, getting help for them will improve your sleep apnea.

- *Adding Oxygen.* Another benefit that can be administered is that of increase oxygen. Your doctor may recommend having you have a supplemental form of oxygen added to your sleep. This will be done in one of various methods, as determined by your condition and by your needs. Here, they will force oxygen into the lungs, keep them full of the air that is required.
- *Positive airway pressure.* This can be needed too. In this case, you may wear what is called a CPAP machine which will force a higher pressured air into your airways. This will keep the airways open and encourage your lungs to have the necessary oxygen that you need.

Those that are suffering from central sleep apnea should take care in what the doctor requires them to do. Although it may seem difficult to wear a mask or it may seem like too much trouble to deal with oxygen at night, it is the difference between life and death in many cases.

Therefore, it is well worth it and in most cases, people will find ways to deal with it so that it becomes no problem at all.

# Learning About Sleep Apnea

Have you been told that you possibly are suffering from sleep apnea? Although this may seem like a very scary situation to be in, many people suffer from it but go on to live very constructive lives. Why is that possible? There are a number of great doctors and procedures that can be done to enhance your quality of life even if you don't realize that you aren't getting what you deserve. Sometimes, the facts are clear that you need help. Other times you may not really know for sure. In any case, if you are having trouble breathing during the night or find yourself unable to sleep soundly, sleep apnea could be to blame for it.

One thing to take note about this condition is that of when it happens. Obstructive sleep apnea is caused by something that is blocking the flow of air freely throughout your body. Your body wants to breath but your actual body is blocking your air way in some way. This is common in people that are overweight or that have large fleshy necks as the skin can cause the airway to become restricted. If you sleep on your stomach at night, this could happen to you as well. This type of apnea happens more often in older adults then it does in younger. It is also twice as commonly found in men as it is found in women.

When it comes to other forms of apnea, the risks are the same. It is important for you to understand what is happening to your body though. Therefore one of the first things that you doctor will recommend is a sleep study. Here, you enter the hospital or lab for an overnight stay. You are monitored while you are sleeping to find out just what is happening to you when you do close your eyes.

You can learn a great deal about sleep apnea if you visit your doctor and talk to your doctor about your condition. If you are looking for the right solution in how to treat it, the first things that need to be done are thorough testing. Once this is done your doctor is likely to recommend the next steps to take to handle it.

# What Are The Symptoms Of Sleep Apnea?

When it comes to sleep apnea, it is something that worries many. The fact is that many people are not sleeping correctly or that they sleep for a full eight hours and wake up feeling as if they didn't sleep at all. Sleep apnea can be the cause of this. More often then not, you won't know that you have this condition but will go to see your doctor because you are just tired all the time. Many people find themselves shocked to hear that something was wrong with their actual sleeping patterns. In fact, many don't realize that anything at all is happening to them.

What are the symptoms that you should look for? No matter what type of sleep apnea that you have, obstructive or central, your symptoms are likely to be about the same. This can make it a bit more difficult to determine what type of apnea you actually suffer from. Here are some of the symptoms that you are likely to be facing.

- **_Hypersomnia_**. You may be tired during the day even though you have slept through the night.
- **_Snoring._** One of the most common symptoms that most people face is that of snoring. There is no doubt that snoring can be tiresome, but it can also be a sign of something much more serious. If your snoring wakes up your spouse, then it is time to talk to your doctor about it.
- **_Morning headaches._** These are another common sign of sleep apnea.

- **_Breathing Cessation._** You may actually observe or notice yourself waking up for no reason in the middle of the night. Or, someone else may notice that you are doing this. Again, your spouse is a great help in spotting this condition.
- **_Dry mouth._** Often, those that suffer from this condition will wake up with the feel of a dry mouth or even a sore throat.
- **_Insomnia._** Many of those that suffer from sleep apnea have insomnia or the condition in which they just can not fall asleep and stay asleep. There may be nothing else causing this to happen. If you wake up with a shortness of breath, it is likely that you will be facing central sleep apnea. If you are more commonly snoring loudly, this is

characterized by obstructive sleep apnea. Nevertheless, if you face any of these problems, it is necessary to talk to your doctor about your condition as soon as possible.

# What Is Causing My Obstructive Sleep Apnea?

Are you having episodes of waking up at night? Is your spouse considering kicking you out of bed because your snoring has gotten so loud? These are signs and symptoms of obstructive sleep apnea. Although it will take a trained doctor to tell you if you do in fact suffer from this condition, it is still something that you may find yourself facing. If and when that happens, it is necessary for you to consider seeking out the help of a doctor to determine what the necessary next step is.

One thing that most that have been told they may have this are wondering is just what is it that causes sleep apnea? There could be several things that cause this condition to effect you.

First of all, the causes for the condition have the same result. In obstructive sleep apnea, the muscles that are located in the very back of your throat relax. What is important to know is that those muscles are actually responsible for supporting the soft palate, the piece of tissue that hangs from the soft palate which is called the uvula and the tonsils and tongue as well.

When this happens to you, your airway is closed off or narrows too much. When you breathe in to take a breath, you can't bring that air into your body and that causes your breathing to stop for that moment. When you miss the breaths that your body requires, your level of oxygen drops considerably and that alarms your brain. To handle this problem the brain tells you to wake up to handle it. In most cases, you will wake up for such a brief second that you don't remember that you even did it.

Sleep apnea of this type of can happen to you over and over again during the night. In some cases it will happen 10, 20 or even 30 times per hour all night long. As you can imagine there is no way for the body to reach deep sleep which is how your body actually rests and becomes recharged. When you can't reach this level of sleep, you probably will wake up and feel as if you didn't sleep at all. Many will find themselves feeling tired during the day too.

# Why Do I Have Central Sleep Apnea?

Central sleep apnea is a condition that many people face and it can be quite alarming. In fact, just being told that you have this condition may be very scary. What do you mean you don't breathe while you are sleeping? That may be what you say right to your doctor. The fact is that during this type of sleep apnea, the conditions are often more serious than with obstructive sleep apnea. In fact, it is often important to realize that if you do have it, it is necessary for you to take actions to correct or manage it successfully.

## What Happens?

During central sleep apnea, your body lacks that effort to breath. Unlike obstructive sleep apnea, the body doesn't have anything that is blocking it from taking air in. In fact, it doesn't have any problems with the airways. Rather, the body has a problem telling itself to breath. Central sleep apnea is much,

much less common then that of obstructive sleep apnea.

In this type of sleep apnea, your brain is where the problem lies. As you know, the brain controls all of the necessary movements and systems in your body. Even when you are sleeping, your brain is working to control things like your breathing. But, when you suffer from central sleep apnea, your brain is making the mistake of not telling your body to breath. Rather, it is not transmitting the necessary signals to your muscles to breath.

When this happens, you wake up feeling like you are out of breath. You may feel like you can't catch your breath. You may face some pretty serious headaches when you awake as well.
There are other symptoms that can be found too, but most often the fact that you remember waking up and feeling as if you can't catch your breath is a warning sign that many doctors take very seriously.

If you have been told that this is a possible cause of your sleeping problems, it is time to talk to your doctor about it. In addition, if you face any of these conditions and remember waking up and experiencing that shortness of breath, it is important that you seek out medical help as these can worsen making sleeping near impossible to do.

# Am I At Risk For Sleep Apnea?

Did you know that many times people can avoid having sleep apnea? If you are someone that experiences shortness of breath when you wake at night, you may actually have a form of sleep apnea is that much rarer called central sleep apnea. This condition is one in which the brain fails to tell your muscles to breath. Nevertheless, the more common type of sleep apnea is that of obstructive sleep apnea. In this situation, individuals have something blocking their air ways and although they are trying to breath, they can't do it.

But, what makes you a candidate for this condition? There are actually several things that could be causing you to face this illness.

• *Overweight.* If you are overweight, excess weight may be playing a role in the problem. If you have extra weight that develops around the upper airway of your body, you may face obstruction in your breathing which can lead to sleep apnea.

Although you may not be overweight, if enough weight develops in this specific area you may be effective (you don't have to look overweight to have to deal with it.)

- **The Size of Your Neck.** Those that have a larger sized neck may also fall victim to sleep apnea. If you have a neck that is larger than 17 inches in its circumference, then you have an increased ability to have sleep apnea.

- **Narrow Airway.** For some people, a narrow airway is just a natural thing and can even be a hereditary condition. In addition, if you have tonsils or adenoids that have become enlarged, you too may be more at risk of developing sleep apnea. These can block the air from flowing easily.

- It is more likely that older people will experience sleep apnea over younger people.

- More men will fall victim to sleep apnea then women will. If you are a woman and are overweight, though, you do have more of a risk than someone that is not overweight.

Sleep apnea is an important condition to have examined. If you have these risk factors and realize that you have some of the symptoms that can lead to sleep apnea, it is essential to talk to your doctor about it. Many times people do not realize that they could be facing a condition that is vitally important to handle.

# Testing For Sleep Apnea

Take a few minutes to find out if you have any of the risk factors or the symptoms of sleep apnea. If you do, contact your doctor to find out what the next step in the process is. One thing that you should realize is that sleep apnea is something that can be hard to diagnose. Yet, it is very important that it is diagnosed successfully. Therefore, you are likely to undergo several different types of treatments to find out if in fact you are suffering from this condition. If in fact you are, then the right steps will be taken to determine just what needs to be done to give you back sleep and return your life to a better quality of life.

There are several tests hat will likely be done on you to determine if you suffer from sleep apnea, what type it is and to what extent you are suffering. In most cases, you will first want to visit a sleep specialist who will handle determining which tests are important for you to take as well as how they will work. In most cases, an overnight evaluation is a must. You will need to monitor how well your breathing is happening during the night as well as your oxygen levels and other body functions.

One of these tests is that of the nocturnal polysomnography. When you have this test, you will have equipment that is placed on you to monitor what is happening with your heart, your brain, and your lungs. It will also look at the breathing patterns that you have during the night. Your arms and legs will be monitored as well. This test is likely to be the first one that you have. It will give the doctor a clear look at if in fact you have sleep apnea.

Two other tests may be needed next. The oximetry test involves just a small device that is fitted over your finger and is completely painless. It will monitor the amount of oxygen in your blood at any time. The portable cardio-respiratory testing device may also be required. Here, you will be able to take the device home with you and it will determine what is happening with your oxygen levels and your breathing while you sleep.

All of these tests are necessary and they are a window into what is happening with your own condition. You will find them to be easy to handle and they give your doctor clear views of what is happening and what to do next.

# What Can Sleep Apnea Do For You?

If you have sleep apnea, you may think that the only thing that can happen to you is that you wake up for no real reason and you find yourself unable to get a good night's sleep. But, this is far from the only thing that can happen to you when you have sleep apnea. In many ways, it can worsen or cause complications that are life threatening. For this reason, if you feel that you may be suffering from this condition, you really should get to a doctor whenever it is possible.

Sleep apnea itself is considered a serious condition that requires help and treatment. There are a number of problems that can come of it. One of the most important things to know is that sleep apnea can cause cardiovascular problems. This is actually due to the low levels of oxygen that you in your blood because your body stops breathing for those seconds. It also increases your blood pressure and therefore strains your heart and the rest of your cardio system. If you have other heart problems, sleep apnea can lead to sudden death that comes from your heart's stopping. If you have central sleep apnea, this actually could be caused by heart disease.

Of course, being tired all day can also be a complication of sleep apnea. If you do anything that requires attention, you may not have enough attention to accomplish the tasks correctly. You may have problems concentrating and problems staying awake. You may also seem to always be in a bad mood because you are irritable.

Other complications that can come of sleep apnea include the fact that you are likely putting yourself at risk if you need to have surgery as anesthesia can be seriously messed up. Of course, most that do in fact have sleep apnea snore quite a bit. This can keep their partners awake during the night keeping them with all the same problems as the other.

As the largest concern of those that suffer from sleep apnea is that of a cardiac event, it is important for you to take head and get to the doctor. It is necessary for you to find out if in fact you have this condition and how you are going to face it. The good news is that those that get help for sleep apnea often sleep the best they have in their lifetime and also have lowered blood pressure because of it.

# Treatments For Obstructive Sleep Apnea

There are many people that face sleep apnea and many of those people don't know it. Yet, even if you don't have any diagnosis of this condition just yet, there is something to look forward to if you do get one. Although sleep apnea is considered a very serious condition and it can leave any number of people at risk for serious health concerns, with treatment the quality of life of that person can be restored in most cases. Sometimes, people get the highest quality of sleep they have gotten for many years. What's more is that it can even help to lower your current blood pressure.

The first types of treatment for a mild to small case of sleep apnea will be to do things to improve your lifestyle. You may be told to stop smoking. You may be instructed to lose weight. These are two of the most common causes of sleep apnea in many people. If you don't get relief from these results, or you have symptoms of a more serious nature, there are a number of treatment options that can in fact work for you.

The CPAP may become your target improvement choice. This is called a continuous positive airway pressure system that will be used while you are sleeping. It is used by people that face both moderate to severe sleep apnea that is caused by an obstruction. The device is actually quite simply a mask that you wear during the night. Although it is not uncomfortable some worry that it will be. What it does is keeps your airways open and that is true benefit to you. To do this, the machine applies a larger amount of air pressure then is in the current air. By doing this, it forces, gently, the airways to stay open, allowing you unrestrictive flow.

Another choice for treating obstructive sleep apnea is to use what is called an oral device. This device is used to keep the breathing airways open while you are sleeping. These are easier to use then the CPAP machine will be, but they don't do as good of a job making it happen.

Finally, in some cases, it may be necessary to have surgery to improve your airway flow. This may or may not be an option for you. One thing to note is that you and your doctor will determine the right method for handling your sleep apnea together and that trial and error may be the best method for improving your quality of life.

# Handling Sleep Apnea

Did you find out that you had sleep apnea? Are you wondering how in the world you are going to deal with this life threatening and troublesome condition? Although sleep apnea is a serious medical condition, there are several methods that can be used to help you to deal with it. The first thing that you need to do is to come to grips with it. Realize that sleep apnea is something that can be handled and in fact many people resolve this problem and get the best sleep of their lifetimes because of it.

Step one in the process of dealing with sleep apnea is education. Your first resource should be your doctor who will explain just what is happening in your situation. Although it may be difficult to realize, he or she is a great person to go to if you want to find out what your possibilities of improving will be. It can also be helpful to learn what the best possible health improvement option is for you.

When it comes to sleep apnea, it is also important to find out if you are getting the best care possible. It is always wise to get a second opinion about your condition and you should never worry about insulting your doctor by doing so. If you are not sure if you should do this or not, the fact that you are questioning it is enough to seek out the help that you need.

Sleep apnea is a serious condition that you have to think about. Each time you go to bed at night, it will be necessary for you to determine if you will get a good night's sleep or if you will allow yourself to suffer because you don't want to seek out the treatment that you deserve.

# Sleep Apnea: When To Get Help

If you are thinking that you may need to seek out the help of your doctor, do so. Sleep apnea is a serious medical condition that can lead to additional compilations as it goes on. In some cases, it will worsen to the point of being something doesn't allow you to sleep and can lead to such serious things as a heart attack. The fight is not worth it, though, as many doctors are well versed in this topic and knows the right methods to handling it.

Nevertheless, you may still not be sure if you need to get help. One sign that you do is if your spouse is complaining about your snoring and just how loud it has gotten. In short, if they can not sleep well because of your snoring, it is time to get help. If you wake up at night and find yourself short of breath and you are not sure why, this can be a sign of a serious issue in that of central sleep apnea. If you find yourself facing pauses in your breathing during your sleep, or your spouse experiences this in you, it is also time to seek out the help you need. Finally, if you get to sleep at night and you just can't understand why you are so tired during the day; this too can be an important consideration.

The fact is that there are countless opportunities that you could be experiencing. One of the most important things for you to do is to recognize the possibility of having something wrong. When this happens to you, or you are considering the fact hat your spouse may have this sleep apnea condition, it is necessary for you to determine the next step that only your doctor will be able to help you with.

# How To Get Quality Care For Sleep Apnea

If you find that you may have some of the symptoms and risks of sleep apnea, it may be necessary to turn to your doctor for help. In fact, if there is any question you should be asking your doctor for help. Yet, there are a number of things to take into consideration when it comes to who to ask and what to say. First and foremost, it is very common for doctors to not be able to diagnosis sleep apnea unless they have had a number of tests done on you. So, your first stop should be with your family doctor to get this Okayed to find a specialist.

Why bother with a specialist in the field? You really do want to find someone that knows what you are facing. You want to find a sleep study clinic, in fact, if that is possible. These can be found in most local areas and are often in hospitals or in other medical facilities that are available around the clock. Because you will need to spend the night here, you will want to make arrangements to not need to be rushed anywhere before or after your come in.

Working with someone that is a specialist means that they are more likely to know how to work the mechanics of the study as well as how to interpret the results effectively.

Those that come in for a sleep study often find themselves unable to sleep. Who can sleep with someone else watching you? Nevertheless, you will want to relax yourself and find a way to get to sleep. It is necessary for you to do this so that they can monitor your condition. In a good facility, they will offer you quiet and will provide a good amount of comfortably that you may not have other places.

# Improving Your Health To
# Avoid Sleep Apnea

If you have any of the risk factors for sleep apnea, you will want to take steps now to reduce those risks significantly. What are those risks? If you are overweight, have a large sized neck or you have enlarged tonsils or a small airway, you are at risk. People that are older than 65 often get this condition and men are more likely to experience it than women are. In addition, those that have heart disease, neurological conditions or other health issues of a serious nature may also have complications from those conditions that can be sleep apnea.

## So, if this is you, what should you do?

•   Don't smoke. Smoking is one of the worst things that you can do for yourself if you do in fact find out that you have sleep apnea. If you have risk factors for it, avoid smoking as this will make the condition that much worse. Smoking reduces the amount of oxygen in your body.

- Lose weight. Maintaining a healthy weight is important. Often, people think that they look fine even though they may have a bit of excess fat around their neck. This is enough to cause a problem for you and it therefore should be treated carefully.

- Monitor your health condition. If you find that you are not getting enough sleep or have any of the symptoms of sleep apnea, get them taken care of as soon as you can. This can prevent them from worsening into a condition that is more life threatening.

## Improving Your Quality Of Life With Sleep Apnea

If you are experiencing sleep apnea and have been diagnosed with it, it is very important for you to seek out the help that you need to keep the condition from getting worse on you. The fact is that whatever the doctor tells you to do is better to just do and deal with then having to face the poor quality living and the risk of a cardiac event that comes from not following doctor's orders. Yet, there are a few things that you can do to help take care of yourself and help allow yourself to get enough rest.

• *Get rid of any excess weight that you can.* Even if you just lose a little amount of weight, you will feel better and may even find that your condition has been lessened considerably.

• *Sleep properly.* That is, make sure that you sleep on your side or on your abdomen instead of sleeping on your back. When you sleep on your back you are more likely to find yourself with additional problems. Although this may be a problem to learn, it will benefit you greatly.

• *Use a saline nasal spray before sleeping.*
This will keep your air ways open while you are
sleeping. You can even get these from your doctor
but before you use them you will want to make sure
that you check with your doctor first.

• *Don't take drugs, alcohol or medications
such as tranquillizers at bed time.* You want
to keep your muscles functioning at their best and
that means not interfering with these things. Each
of them will cause the muscles in your throat to
become looser then they should be.

If you suffer from sleep apnea, it is essential to
seek out the help of a qualified doctor. Once you
get a treatment program in place, you can find
real benefits in improving your health and well
being. It is worth it.

# Pick A Pillow To Help Stop Snoring

We've all heard the argument that if you elbow a snorer and they roll over, their snoring will stop. In some cases this actually works and after rolling over, the snorer and the person doing the elbowing both get a good and quiet night's rest.

There are devices that you can purchase that help the snorer to sleep in a position that encourages less snoring. The idea behind them is that if the snorer's body is in a certain position the airway through their throat will be more open and that allows a clearer passage of air. The more air that gets through, the less likely the person is to snore.

For some people it might mean lying on their side with two or three pillows under their head. In this case it's just about experimenting with the number of pillows and adjusting them so that the snorer is not only comfortable but the snoring stops.

There are specialty pillows that can be purchased that create a contour under the neck of the person who snores. This contour works as a method of opening up the throat and generally they are designed to aid the snoring problem regardless of which position the snorer sleeps in, whether it's his or her back or side. These can be quite costly so it's important to research them before investing in one.

Another overlooked aspect of pillows is that they can contain products that the snorer might be allergic to. This results in an accumulation of mucous in the person's throat which results in their snoring. Not connecting the two can lead to years of snoring problems without recognizing that the pillow is the culprit. By changing to a pillow made with another material, the snoring may stop.

# Nose Strips: Can They Help Stop Snoring?

Within the past few years the problem of snoring has become more of an issue. People are discussing it more and researchers are trying to come up with new and inventive ways for dealing with the problem.

One of those new ideas involves the use of strips that adhere to the skin of the nose. They are found under various brand names, but their goal is common, and that goal is to stop snoring.

The premise for how they work is that the snorer applies an adhesive strip to their nose. It lays across the bridge of their nose in a horizontal fashion. At first glance it resemblances the type of adhesive strip that a person would use to cover a cut or a scrape. But instead of the strips designed for snoring is a narrow thick material when applied helps to open the nostrils. The idea is that when the nose is held open the person it is applied to will not snore because they are able to breathe without obstruction.

The strips are discreet in that they are not applied until the person is going to bed. They don't need to be worn during the day and they rarely cause an allergic reaction so it's not obvious to anyone that you have worn them.

They are effective in many people. People claim that by using the strips, their snoring has stopped completely. They have found relief in one of the most natural ways possible without consuming any medications at all.

If you snore or you live with a snorer, buying a package of these types of snoring aids might just bring the type of relief from snoring you've been searching for. They aren't that expensive and they are certainly well worth the cost of a good night's sleep.

# Sing Your Way To A Silent Night

We've all been guilty of it. Driving down the road while a song plays from the radio, we sing along not even sure if we know the words. Its fun, it's relaxing and it might also be a great way to stop snoring.

When a person sings they are in essence exercising the muscles of their throats. We use those muscles each day while we talk but they get a more extensive work out when a person sings.
These are the same muscles that are used when a person snores.

If those muscles weaken a bit we might be more prone to snoring. Snoring is at the very least a very large inconvenience, and having a solution that is fun and entertaining would make the problem much easier to deal with.

If you do suffer from snoring than it might be time to tune up your voice and pick a favorite song or two to sing to. This doesn't have to be done in front of others if you are uncomfortable with your singing voice. It can be done while you are home alone or in your vehicle as you drive to work. A few moments, once or twice a day may be the difference between a night filled with snoring and one filled with silence.

A few suggestions for using singing as a snoring solution are:

- Pick a song you are familiar with. Trying to sing to something new will not only be frustrating but difficult on your voice.
- Pick a song that has an easy to follow melody.
- Vary the choice of songs so you don't become bored of the exercise.
- Sing in the shower if you can, the steam will help lubricate your throat muscles which also helps with snoring.

You don't have to become the next platinum recording artist, but if singing can stop your snoring, it might be time move from lip synching to actual singing.

# Can Acupressure Help Stop Snoring?

For centuries people have sought aid for many ailments in the process of acupressure. It is used to treat everything from headaches to being an aid in weight loss. Acupressure has proven results and it also has proven that it can help stop snoring.

The key to acupressure as a snoring cure can be found in your little finger. It is thought that by applying pressure to your little finger, the mechanisms that cause snoring aren't triggered.

There are a couple of different approaches to this technique. One is to visit someone who is experienced in the art of acupressure. You will discuss your snoring problem with them and they will explain the process and the benefits as they relate to you. By using pressure on certain points of your body they can help energy to flow in a specific way throughout your body. This can greatly influence whether or not you snore.

Another choice is to wear a device that produces

pressure on your little finger throughout the night. One of the devices that is available on the market today is a bracelet. It is designed to be worn while a person is asleep and it's believed to stop snoring by keeping a constant amount of pressure on the finger allowing the energy in the body to flow in such a manner that snoring ceases.

For people who have used acupressure in the past to deal with health issues, using it as a means to end snoring is a great alternative. They are familiar with the procedures and results that can be achieved. For those new to the idea of acupressure, if they are leaning towards it as a way to end their nights of snoring, it's a wonderful way to be introduced to what acupressure has to offer.

## Beware: Sleeping Pills Can Actually Worsen Snoring

For someone who has difficulty sleeping, having a sleep aid such as a sleeping pill can seem almost a lifesaver. If a person has slept restlessly for months or even years, being able to take something and then fall into a deep sleep can seem like a wonderful solution.

That deep sleep might also result in snoring. For those around the person sleeping away under the influence of a sleeping pill, it can mean a night without any sleep at all.

When we take a sleeping aid, our body relaxes to a point that we feel exhausted and naturally drift off to sleep. Our throat muscles become relaxed at the same time and this can result in snoring. Stopping the snoring might mean stopping the sleeping aid.

Often when a person is having difficulty sleeping they attribute that to stress or being overworked. The problem might be right in front of their eyes though. The problem might be that because of their snoring, they aren't sleeping. When they take a sleeping aid the snoring problem just worsens.

Their body is so relaxed and they are in such a deep sleep that the snoring can actually become dangerous and be a symptom of sleep apnea which is when the person stops breathing.
Therefore it's important to recognize that although the sleeping aid is beneficial it might also be damaging to the snorer.

In this case, when the person does have a snoring problem, it's important to find the cause of the snoring, whether that's being overweight, being allergic to something or sleeping in the wrong position. Although sleeping pills might help the snorer get a great night's rest, others will feel the opposite and long for a peaceful sleep free of the sounds of snoring.

# Causes Of Snoring In Children

It might not be an abnormal occurrence for children to snore, since about 12 percent of them snore from one year to nine years. But, if your child is snoring, do not take it for granted, you should take that child for medical examination to actually determine the cause of snoring as to certify the safe health of the child.

If your child snores consistently, it might be a result of OSAS known as sleep apnea syndrome. In this case, the child's snore might be very loud and he or she is usually restless through the night because of the uncomfortable breathing conditions. This will lead to the child waking up several times at night, and each time he or she returns to sleep, the loud snore continues immediately. This is not a usual occurrence for most children, but every parent must be aware of some of the factors that might indicate the existence of the sleep apnea (OSAS).

Most of the factors that indicate this condition are:

The lack of the ability to pronounce words perfectly. The child will experience a speech impediment making it difficult to speak clearly. The child will experience retardation in growth since all his or her energy is used up while breathing. This also makes it difficult for the child to eat well, because of the struggle to breathe and eat at the very same time - this makes the feeding time a very slow process.

Because of lack of proper sleep the child experiences the feeling of drowsiness and in the effort to be alert hyperactivity becomes the end point. It will be discovered that the child educational performance in school is not good, because of the lack of peaceful sleep at night.

If you notice these signs in your child, it will probably mean he or she has a sleep apnea and in that case, a visit to the pediatric doctor will be recommended as this issue will be analyzed with medical examinations to get a treatment suitable for the child. When treated the child's performance at school will improve since sufficient sleep is denied at night.

There are also other factors that cause snoring in children apart from sleep apnea (OSAS), and they are:

Children suffering from asthmatic conditions snores, because this ailment affects the respiratory system, thus producing snoring while the child sleeps.

When the adenoids of a child is enlarged as a result of the infiltrations of allergies bringing about the inflammation of nasal linings, the child snores. This is because the breathing process of the child is impaired and every thing returns back to normal once the allergy is treated.

Children suffering from obesity will also snore, statistics show that about 40 percent children suffering from obesity snores. In this case, there are obstructions produced in the respiratory pathways of air as a result of the accumulation of fat round about the throat region. Too much fat can also result to the malfunctioning of the diaphragm which can also result to snoring.

When a child experiences cold, the organs in the

nasal and respiratory cavities are enlarged leading to snoring. If the adenoid is enlarged it can also cause snoring. These two conditions if treated will bring about the end to the snoring sound produced by the child while sleeping.

Other instances like the inability of the muscles and nerves of the child to handle the movement of the air passages in the respiratory tract can lead to snoring. When the child's jaw was not properly developed, snoring can be the resultant problem.

# Factors that Cause Snoring

There are in reality so many factors that leads to snoring and most of these factors vary from person to person; however, there are some major root causes of snoring. Snoring is the noisy disturbance produced by the movements of airflow during sleep. It is the noise emitted when there is a restriction experienced in the out flow and in flow of air in the respiratory passages.

It has been observed that this noise called snoring is usually experienced only during sleep. This makes me wonder why the noise is only made when an individual is asleep. If one will snore, why not during ant time of the day, especially when awake, but this is not possible, because the snoring sound is a product of muscles that are relaxed and inactive. When the respiratory muscles are active, there can not be snoring.

The vibration occurs only during sleep, because of the softness of the different parts of the respiratory system at the point of sleep, all these organs are relaxed, hence the noise of snoring becomes obvious. There are different types of snores as a result of the disparity in the level of sounds produced varying from one person to another. The level of the produced sound is directly proportional to the level of strength with which the air passing through the respiratory passages. If the air passage is very forceful, then, the sound of the snore be very high and vice versa. In this case even a baby can snore, but the sound produced in this case is very mild and makes no visible difference, since the air passes with very little force or strength.

The act of snoring while sleeping is common to both men and women at all ages, but studies have proved that men of middle ages are more prone to the attack of snoring than others. In general men are more affected by snoring than women, because of the differences in the structure of the neck. The neck of a man is larger than that of a woman and other organs in the respiratory system differs, leading to the sexual disparity in snoring. This in conjunction with the fact that the forcefulness of air passages are higher in men than in women.

Furthermore, the production of the birth hormones called progesterone in women also makes them less prone to snoring, because these hormones produced during pregnancy and lactation prevents snoring since it gives remedy to the act of snoring. It has also been discovered that some devices to stop snoring actually contain these hormones as an antidote to snoring.

Apart from these above mentioned, some other factors below can cause snoring:

1. If someone is obsessed, snoring can not be avoided.
2. Drunkenness can also cause snoring.
3. If you are experiencing flu with cold, the nasal passages might be blocked leading to snoring.
4. Other factors can also block the air passages such as allergies leading to snoring.
5. Some drugs can dry up the nasal passages.
6. The cavities of the nose can thicken resulting to snoring
7. If you have a large belly, snoring is un avoided.

8. With a tongue that is large, the respiration will be blocked causing snoring.

9. If you use too much sprays nasally, snoring occurs.

10. Smoking of cigarettes leads to inflamed air paths causing snoring.

# Top Anti Snoring Devices You Can Avail

It is not in any way interesting to be in the same room with a person that snores, the level of closeness or the amount of love shared between the two parties becomes insignificant when it comes to dealing face to face with snoring. It does not matter if the person snoring is your mother, spouse, friend or even the love of your life - it is very annoying and irritating to sleep in the same bedroom with a snorer. In fact, I can not stand being in the same house with such an individual.

Through the intervention of scientists that are carrying out unending researches to eradicate the snoring habit, some devices have been produced to help snorers all over the world. And some of the best devices to stop snoring are listed below:

## Nasal Dilators

This is a device used to open up the passages through which air enters and flows out of the nose. it is fabricated from either plastic or coil of stainless steel.

## Pillows to Stop Snoring

These are special pillows produced to help the snorer position himself or herself rightly so as to avoid snoring. When an individual sleeps in the wrong position, the out flow and in flow of air through the respiratory tract is hampered or restricted bringing about snoring. So, the pillow is designed to solve this problem.

## Snore Balls

To a snorer, it is very important to have the right sleeping posture and the best position to sleep is by the sides. When someone prone to snoring sleeps on his or her back there is always an increased tendency to snore while sleeping. This is the actual reason for the snore balls; a tennis ball, golf ball, or even a base ball can be used. All you need to do is place it at the back, so that whenever you try to sleep on your back, the sharp pain experienced will make you do otherwise; causing you to remain on your sides. This is painful but very effecti

## Nasal Strips

These are strips put into the nose to keep the flow of air constant. In this case there is a free constant flow of air through the nose to every part of the respiratory organ making it easy to breathe, hence there will be no snoring. This device is also utilized by athletes during exercises or competitions.

## Throat Spray

The throat spray is a combination of natural components mixed to produce a special spray which the snorer can use before sleeping on his or her throat to eradicate snoring. But one has to be very careful about the throat spray since an excessive use of it can cause more harm than good.

## Sleep Position Monitor

It is very clear that to stop snoring, a person must always adopt the habit of sleeping in the right position. If this is not adhered to the habit can not be eradicated. The best sleeping position is by the sides. The sleep posture monitor releases a sharp beep whenever the person attempts to sleep in the wrong position. This instrument is not the best choice, especially if the person trying to stop snoring does not live alone, because the beeps will disturb his or her room mate.

Apart from the natural factors like sleeping position or restricted air flow through the respiratory tract; there are other factors that causes snoring medically, so, the best option is to carry out a medical examination first before choosing the method of treatment. What ever treatment is prescribed, follow the prescription strictly and the snoring will be overcome.

## A Change In Lifestyle Is A Good Remedy To Stop Snoring

Its been proven that approximately 45 percent Americans snore often. And its shocking to know that almost 80 percent of them sleep in different rooms, and even worse is to know that couples have actually divorced, thanks to snoring.

Snoring creates some sort of stress in a relationship, and also a complex of a different sort. This does not just affect your partner, but also you, just think, in spite of all the beauty, if one snores during their sleep, it will be awful, not just for them, but for people around also.

It would be really funny to think, but, would the prince who was supposed to kiss the sleeping beauty kissed her in case she was sleeping with the company of loud snores?

That might be something funny to think about, on a larger scale and a wider perspective, the social consequences that arise due to snoring are a lot. The snoring might gradually lead to mild sleep apnea, which is a dangerous disorder, where your breathing halts for a good 60 second gap. So, snoring must not be pushed aside thinking that its some simple thing.

Snoring can lead to diabetes, unbelievable, isn't it? That is what is up for us in the recent surveys. The logic behind this is simple, snoring cuts down the intake of oxygen, which leads to a situation where a lot of catecholamines are produced. Thus, you can be attacked by diabetes.

Before we hit the treatments to prevent snoring, let us discuss about the root cause that leads to snoring. How many of us have questioned as to why people snore? The answer is here, when we sleep, the air passing through our nose then to the throat and then to the lungs move noiselessly, but for many people, there might be some sort of obstruction in the air flow. The reasons might be clogged nose or something else, but whatever it is, it just hampers the airflow.

Usually, snoring is caused by the tissue that is soft, in the throat, which vibrates, thus, the airway is clogged, and it passes to the lungs, and it creates a noise. The snoring is due to the air passing across the tissue there.

Now, coming to the prevention of snoring. How is it possible?

There is no readymade answer for this, but there are a lot of solutions for people who are disheartened by the way they snore. Let us focus on the lifestyle, and the possible ways in which it can worsen the snoring problem, and also the ways in which lifestyle can cure snoring.

Anything done in excess, like, smoking, drinking, eating, are all things that can make this problem worse. And not doing these are methods by which one can prevent snoring, before leaping to other hard attempts to prevent snoring, like surgery.

A good guide to follow, in case snoring is to be prevented:


· 	Never take too much of food before you crash, take a good three hour rest before going to sleep, and after taking your final meal.

- A balanced diet is another thing that is important to keep snoring at bay.

- Burning the excess calories by exercising is another important thing.

- Allergies are to be checked by keeping the surroundings clean.

- Never leave the window open when you sleep.

- Fatigue must be prevented, and a normal sleep

# Causes Of Snoring And Finding Treatment Through Surgery

One of the greatest problems and one of the most common one during sleep is snoring. Its not as bad as dying, but still, snoring sure has its own problems tagged along, that are really grave. There are many other problems that might root from snoring.

This is a common phenomenon in men who are classified in the middle age, and more with the men who are obese. This has a probability with fat men, as they have enlarged and flesh filled throats, whose muscles might collapse when relaxed.

Snoring has its roots from the airflow in the passage that is between the nose and the throat. The relaxation of tissues will only make the passage more narrow. This is the possible answer for people asking why we snore only when we are relaxed.

The airflow in the narrow air passage along the relaxed muscles in the throat invariable initiate a vibration. The muscle relaxes and the tongue falls back and waits for the muscle to be relieved off the tension that is thrown on it.

A blocked nose can also contribute to this situation, as the space in the nose becomes limited and less air passes through, so, sometimes, the snoring occurs only when a person has heavy cold, or profound sinus.

Snoring can be an effect of the position in which one person sleeps, if he sleeps on his back, then, the tongue naturally falls back , and the throat muscles are pulled by gravity. So, people are generally suggested to sleep in the sideward position.

The relaxation of muscles in the throat is the culprit, it is unwanted and this causes the airflow to get lessened and the respiratory tract and the nasal paths are troubled, so, its better to get the excess muscles fixed.

The real cause for the snoring is only found when an otolaryngologist inspects it. The specialist will surely be able to find the reason, and the other problems related to the ear, the nose and the throat.

The surgery conducted on you to stop snoring is called the uvulopalatoharyngoplasty, acronym as UPPP, it is just widening the passages for airflow. This process removes the tissues that are excessive in the throat and that narrows down the passage.

A more intensive one is the Laser uvulopalatoharyngoplasty.

Both are done on mild snorers, but don't have the desired effect with people suffering from apnea.

Nasal surgery is one way to help people from snoring, and it is recommended to people whose nasal septum is blocked.

There is another method where the tongue is kept from falling back, and it is called to Tongue Suspension Procedure. Here, the tongue is stitched below with the lower jaw with the help of a small screw.

The throat tissue plays a major role in snoring, so shrinking it will ultimately give you a solution. The name of the method to shrink your excess tissue in the throat by releasing energy with the help of electrode needles is called Somnoplasty. This, later is absorbed back by the body.

Surgery is not one of the most preferred and the simplest ways of fixing the sloppy throat muscles. But it sure is the ultimate solution to snoring. But, it is best to discuss this with the physician, and he will give the best method to help you from snoring.

# Snoring Cure: What Are They?

You might find people who snore funny, but you just won't feel the same way when the person you sleep with snores into your ear every night. It in fact will annoy you. This is the driving force behind curing snoring.

The following are some methods to control or if possible cure snoring:

1. **Respiratory Exercises**: Snoring is mainly caused by blocks in the breathing passage like the nose and throat due to nose blockades, wrongly position jaws or an over-strained throat. To resume normal breathing, take many deep breaths to relax the muscles of your throat

2. **Decongestants**: Nasal congestion can also cause snoring. Since the nose is blocked, the person may try to breathe through the mouth leading to snoring. To clear these blockades, take decongestants.

**3. *Anti-allergy medications***: Enlargement of adenoids might have been cause by allergy to some drug previously prescribed. Once a person gets over the allergy, snoring stops.

**4. *Healthy diet and exercise***: Most obese people snore. This is not just a coincidence. The concentration of fat in the air passage, limits air from flowing freely in and out. The proper functioning of the diaphragm is also hindered by fat accumulation in the stomach resulting in snoring. 4 in 10 obese people are known to snore. Good exercise and a healthy diet will not alone help them overcome snoring, but will also benefit them in numerous ways.

**5. *Change your bed position***: Sleeping in the wrong position may also induce snoring. For example, you might stretch your neck too much by using too many pillows. Using a single pillow can avoid this. Lying on your back may also cause snoring.

**6. *Lifestyle change***: Intake of alcohol and snoring may directly or indirectly induce snoring. For example, certain medical complications caused by drinking might have caused snoring. To maintain good health, it is therefore advisable to quit alcohol and smoking. This also improves all-round health and mental peace.

7. **Medication**: Sleeping pills, antihistamines, certain other medicines can cause an increase in snoring.

8. **Sleep Pattern:** Basically, there are two periods of sleep, the REM sleep and stage 1 sleep. A person dreams constantly in REM sleep and experiences deep sleep often. Stage1 sleep will be experienced while sleeping or if a person sleeps poorly. Both these can lead to unstable breathing which in turn causes snoring. If you don't sleep at around the same time everyday, the irregularity may cause instability in respiration and thus cause unstable breathing when you sleep.

9. **Salt water nasal drops**: Congestion in the nose may be caused by mucus and this can both spoil your sleep and also cause snoring. If you want to avoid this, purchase a small bottle of salt water nasal drops at any drugstore in your neighborhood. These help flush down the mucus. If you are not willing to buy a bottle, these nasal drops can be made right at home

by dissolving a teaspoon of salt in roughly 250 ml of water. Once this water cools to the natural temperature of the body, put a dripper in it and use it.

If any other serious condition like sleep apnea or enlargement of tonsils and/or adenoids, surgical procedures such as Laser Assisted Uvula Palatopathy commonly abbreviated as LAUP and somnoplasty or radio frequency tissue ablation can be undertaken. This is more than sufficient proof that the root cause of snoring must be determined prior to taking action.

# Free Yourself From Snoring: Simple Home Remedies To Stop Snoring

Do you often find your spouse sleeping in a different room? If the answer is yes, then the most likely reason is the annoying melodies produced by you when asleep. You might be able to sleep well with this music, but it can make your spouse pull out his/her hair in bunches.

Wondering what is being referred to as music here? In lay man's terms, it is called snoring. The only instrument you need to play it is your own throat. Though it is common, it can be disastrous to relationships. It has driven some people to the extent of taking a divorce on grounds of snoring.

This is an indication of a malfunction in your body. Many people who have studied snoring in depth have found that it may be a sign of diabetes of obesity or something much more serious like a serious heart condition that has gone undiagnosed.

Not alone is your partner's sleep affected, but even

you will often have to turn and find a better sleeping position to avoid snoring. All this might be done by you thoroughly unaware that it was snoring that woke you up in the first place. The most vital organ of the human body, the brain, need a constant supply of sufficient oxygen to prevent damage to itself. Snoring occurs only when you obstruct your own windpipe. Thus the brain gets alerted and wakes you up from deep slumber to open up the blocked air passage. You may not even know that you had woken up.

But your partner who lost her sleep would watch the entire event.

Snoring leads to various complications like lack of sleep, headaches right in the morning, irritability, lightheadedness etc and spoils your entire day. Now that you know the various ill- effects of snoring and have realized that it is not to be ignored, let us look at some simple but effective cures for it.

To treat snoring, first we have to know the cause. The chief cause of snoring is relaxation of throat muscles. These tend to relax when you are sleeping, and if they are too relaxed because of fatty tissues, they will obstruct the passage of air to the lungs. Air that is moving in and out, makes these fatty tissues and throat muscles vibrate, which produces the annoying sound.

So we have zeroed down on the cause. Let us find a cure for it.

Being overweight is one of the main causes of snoring. Sagging of throat muscles is caused by the fat tissues that build up around it. So the simplest way to prevent snoring is to monitor your weight. Consume a healthy and balanced diet and exercise to keep the muscles toned. After a certain stage, you will finally stop snoring or at least reduce it to a tolerable level to satisfy both your spouse and you.

The following are some other remedies for snoring that can be practiced from home.

1. ***Do not smoke*** - These tend to make your throat muscles relax a bit too much

2. ***Do not consume alcoholic beverages*** - They too tend to over-relax your throat muscles.

3. ***Eat light and healthy*** - Heavy dinner causes sagging of throat muscles

4. ***Do not take sedatives*** - Throat muscles relax more than required.

5. ***Don't lie on your back*** - Moderate snorers stop snoring when lying on their sides.

6. ***Get a small comfortable pillow*** - Large pillows feel comfortable but increase tendency to snore

7. ***Elevate your bed*** - Inclining your bed to a small angle with the upper torso elevated is effective in checking snoring. You can elevate it with a pair of old hard-bound books.

That is it. They might sound simple and easy to practice. But they work wonders in curing snoring. Have a good night's sleep.

## Slip Away From Snoring By Using Herbal Remedy

Many new drugs have come out into the mainstream market which claim to reduce drastically if not completely cure snoring. For those few for whom all these medicines have failed, doctors suggest surgery as the drastic last resort.

But what do you do, if you thoroughly dislike medicines and are scared of the knife. Are you doomed to be the laughing stock for snoring for the rest of your life?

This can probably drive you nuts if you were unaware that herbs are very effective in curing snoring. No. This is not a mere sales gimmick. You can stop snoring through herbal cures. Of the various methods to prevent or completely stop snoring that are out there today, you must agree that natural supplements are much safer than drugs which are normally prescribed.

Please note that natural is not synonymous with without recommendation. There are certain natural substances that can hamper the course of action of other drugs and need to be avoided since they can be intoxicating.

Advice of a medical expert must be sought before administering any of these supplements. Else, conduct researches yourself.

This is more strongly advice if you are already under medication or are allergic to certain things that can be triggered by these supplements. Much like their artificial counterparts, even herbal drugs must be taken only in carefully prescribed doses.

There are people who have an aversion to taking artificial medicines and believe that natural supplements are the way to go to gracefully treat the human body.

It is because of this that knowledge of natural alternatives to cure snoring is sought after. A large portion of people will prefer it over even medicines that are readily available in the market and have natural ingredients.

Aromatherapy is another well-known cure for snoring. This method uses certain oils to relax the airway. The anti-inflammatory action of these oils is taken advantage of here. You may also use these oils through sprays or mouth rinses.

Though this method is simple, it is strongly discouraged for people with asthma or any previous breathing problems. Avoid contact with eyes. Consult a doctor immediately if it accidentally falls into the eyes.

Herbal supplements packaged in the form of tablets are also widely used. These help clearing mucus in the throat and helps relaxing the air pipe. Mucous causes blocking of the insides of the throat which is normally ignored by the person who snores. This produces a contraction of the windpipe which further leads to snoring. These tablets help alleviate these problems.

Hungry for more information on this interesting cure? Search engines can be your friend and guide in this venture. Search for then with apt keywords like "Herbal snoring cure" or "Natural cure for snoring" to find millions of pages on the topic.

A homeopathic professional is best suited to suggest what you can take and what you must avoid.

There are thousands of success stories where people have successfully overcome snoring. Try it yourself and join them.

A word of caution: What may suit others may not suit you. One man's food is another's poison.

# Apt To The Body, Apt To The Purse: The Affordable Herbal Snoring Remedy

The prospect of curing snoring through herbs is spreading like wildfire throughout the world. This is probably because these remedies are more gentle on the human body than normal drugs.

These medicines not alone cure snoring, but also are way cheaper than artificial medicines. People tend to relate herbal medicines to China because of their extensive knowledge of herbs. Snoring, after probably common cold, is something that troubles almost everybody. If frequent snorers feel doomed to snoring, even people who snore irregularly have disturbed sleep patterns due to it. This sound that comes out through the mouth while sleeping can be really embarrassing and disturbing.

Snoring not alone disturbs the snorer, but also the people who share the bed with them. People have gone to the extent of commenting that it is a nightmare to sleep with a snorer. Snoring may also be the indication of cardiac problems or hypertension. So don't you dare take it lightly.

At the same time however, you need not worry too much. There are a wide range of drugs and devices that are available at almost every pharmacy to relieve you of this predicament. These may be good, but herbal remedies have of late proven to be more effective and cheap.

These medicines cure snoring, widen the air passage and give you a good night's rest. Note that people who are already under allopathic medication for snoring shouldn't immediately switch to herbal remedies. One must consult his/her physician first to make sure that one would not have side-effects.

Herbs unlike normal drugs also improve your overall health. They set right imbalance in the body an also improve the immune system. your energy will also be increased and you will lead a whole new lease of life.

Using herbs is very specific to your symptoms and each of these medicines is taken from a different source and hence have varied indications and actions on the body.

China has been the early bird in herbal cures and has been practicing it for centuries. This is enough proof that it is safe to use. It is free from all side-effects that could normally arise. Still, to reap maximum benefit from them, an herbalist's advice is suggested.

The biggest advantage of these cures is that it restores balance in the body. It treats only the part where it is supposed to act on leaving the rest of the body untouched. Man becomes ill only when his body's balance is disturbed.

A second advantage of these natural cures is that it is suite for each person's specific needs. Therefore, when buying herbal drugs, approach companies that take custom orders. Pre- packaged doses may be a bit cheaper but also a tad less effective. There are many such companies that produce even single-order medicines.

Many herbal medicines that have been developed recently don't even need cooking. Herbal medicines come in diverse forms ranging from tablets to oral solutions, pills to powders, spray to lotion to liniments or even as a tea bag! You can take them in whichever form is comfortable to you. The effectiveness of each of these is different.

For those who monitor their cash stringently, these medicines are a blessing compared to their costlier European alternatives. Therefore use herbal medicines if you wish to remain at the pink of your health. It not alone cures snoring but also relieves you of the hassles of side-effects.

# Home Remedies For Snoring People, Why Not?

Are you one of those who experience sleepless nights because your partner snores non-stop? Or are you the person who is snoring and wants to get over it, the cost-effective way? Get that odd noise out of your household today. Here are some simple cures for snoring.

To find a cure for snoring, we need to zero down on its cause. Research shows that snoring or stertor as it is medically referred to is cause by air vibration when it is forced through a small gap inside the throat which is stuffed.

Did you wonder why we tend to snore only when we are sleeping? When we sleep, our upper airway muscles relax and they wilt inward. This makes passage of air through the wind pipe tougher and hence apnea (stoppage of breathing of small instants)occurs which leads to snoring

When apnea occurs, there is an increase in Carbon

dioxide levels in the body. In response to this, the heart rate gets affected and our blood vessels get narrowed. Thus the more time for which these muscles relax, the more the people snore. There are people who do not realize that they are snoring. They toss and turn and wake up tired losing good quality sleep. Some people, when half-awake, even hear themselves snoring.
Obesity, smoking, drinking, tonsillitis, sinusitis, common cold may all lead to snoring.

Snoring is closely linked to overweight people. This is because there is fat concentration on the airways that limits the air to go in and out freely. Losing weight will greatly help these people to stop snoring.

Consume healthy food and exercise everyday. Though it may seem unrelated, exercising is found to be very effective in getting rid of snoring. A relaxed jaw can work wonders in reducing snoring.

If you do smoke or drink, reduce their frequency. By minimizing consumption of alcohol during the night, you can overcome snoring and you will also experience a complete improvement in health. Research shows that bad sleeping positions can cause snoring. Lying on your back may cause snoring. So lying on your stomach or to your sides may help you overcome snoring.

Soreness of the upper respiratory tract, Nose blocks and tonsillitis are the chief causes of snoring in young children. Children, and even adults for that matter, tend to breathe with their mouth when their nose is blocked. This as expected leads to snoring. So if you started snoring because of cold, the snoring will also go away when you are rid of cold. That is it. Cure snoring through the above means. Curing it is necessary since it reflects on our mood and our relationship with others.

Though these remedies may cure the woes of most of those who snore, they are not a panacea. They can most certainly reduce snoring, but it may not completely cure it. Medicines or sprays that are get at pharmacies to cure snoring are too at times ineffective. So it is better to take these home-remedies and not have anything to lose.

## Ways To Prevent The Causes
## Of Snoring

Snoring is way too common. But does this mean you can ignore it? Many do, but let us see why snoring is not insignificant.

It is caused by air striking loose tissues in the neck. When the entire body relaxes, even these muscles tend to relax and they cause a person to snore. If you ever wondered why we snore only when we are asleep, this would have answered your question. When you are awake, these muscles are taut and so air flows through freely. But when you sleep, they tend to droop and thus we snore.

When the tongue falls back into the throat, the pressure in the throat is increased exponentially leading to difficulty in passage of air. So air cannot flow like it did before. When the air passing strikes the back of the tongue, the tongue vibrates producing the drumming sound labeled by us as the snore.

People who approach physicians for curing snoring

are often asked to lie on their sides since lying on their back can lead to excess relaxation of neck muscles effectively cutting down the amount of air that passes. Gravity will cause these tissues to dangle and the tongue to roll back into the throat. This leads to snoring.

One of the earliest and simplest devices to keep a person from snoring is a tennis ball stitched inside a sock attached to the back of a snorer's pajama. This restricts a person from lying on his back. So he sleeps on his side instead and relieves himself of the snore.

The most common victims of snoring are the obese. There are far more loose, flabby tissues in their neck and this forms a greater barrier to the flow of air leading to snoring. The loudness of one's snore is often proportional to the amount of excess fat one has.

The best way to prevent snoring is to keep your weight under check. Not alone will you avoid snoring but you will also he saved from various cardiac diseases, impairments and you will start feeling more confident

Choose the best way to lose weight. This could be gymming or a jog or yoga. Don't rush it up. Rome was not built in a day. So weight accumulated gradually will be lost gradually. Speeding it up can lead to adverse results. Keep exercising and also stick to a strict diet. It will pay ten fold.

Substances that induce relaxation can also trigger snores. Do not consume Do not get too tired on any given day. Work within your limits, else you may relax too much leading to snoring.

Sleep at around the same time everyday. When the body gets used to this, it relaxes more and this gives you better sleep. Thus even if your snoring disturbs your partner, you are less likely to be awakened by this annoying grunt.

Breathing through the mouth is quite often the cause of snoring since the dropped jaws tend to make the tongue dangle into the throat. So you have to overcome it. This can be done by practicing nasal breathing as soon as you realized that you are breathing through your mouth. This is not something very difficult since any treatment for snoring involves switching to nasal breathing from using your mouth. Prevention is clearly better than cure when it comes to snoring.

# Want To Quit Snoring? Know What Causes The Problem

Snoring, undeniable worsens your health and strains relationships. There is no wonder then why too many people want to quit snoring. Also everybody needs some rest after a hectic day.

The really sad thing is snoring is not voluntary. In fact, most smokers are blissfully unaware of snoring until they are told that they snore by their partners. These people can either control their throat muscles from dangling loosely or they can initiate snoring.

It is very hard to find the correct cause of snoring because there a myriad reasons that contribute to it. Man has however devised various methods to locate the culprit. It is well known in the field of medicine that a cure can be easily found for a symptom whose cause is found. It is therefore quintessential for a person to find out the one reason that is actually aggravating his snoring.

Any problem is incurable only when its root can't

be identified. There are many reasons as to why a person snores. When we zero down on the right one, we can cure it with ease. But locating the cause has itself proven to be time consuming.

It all comes down to you realizing what went wrong. So if you identify the trigger for your problems, you can overcome it.

Smokers are found to have a greater chance to start snoring than non-smokers. Smoking is linked with way too many health hazards that can even prove life-threatening and fatal. Snoring is not fatal, but it can cause a lot of discomfort and losing sleep can indirectly lead to hypertension and cardiac problems. It makes you lose certain specific pleasures too.

The smoke and the substances in the cigarette smoke cause the esophagus's cells to react. Thus a chain reaction sets up in a smoker's throat and lungs that cause secretion of extra mucus to enable the lining to withstand the new harsh conditions. This leads to the accumulation of unwanted substances in your air passage which prevents free flow of air in and out of the lungs. This wildly aggravates snoring.

If you smoke, it might be the cause of you snoring. To make sure if this is the cause of you snoring, quit snoring for some time, and see the miraculous changes yourself.

Consumption of alcohol goes to the negative extreme. When a person drinks before sleeping, the neck muscles relax a bit too much. Once these muscles are relaxed in excess, they tend to slump into the free spaces in your throat. This leads of obstruction of air. When these muscles vibrate with flow of air, snoring occurs.

The obese are more prone to start snoring than those who have their weight under control. The heavier a person becomes, greater are the chances that he will start snoring when he is asleep. Snoring doesn't start only because the person is obese. The likelihood increases because when a person becomes fatter, he will have more tissues in the airway in his neck.

Since these tissues obstruct normal flow of breath, snoring might occur. A few others start snoring because of some form of allergy.

There are a dozen other reasons to why you snore. The only way to find out is to devise ways to find out! A general physician might be able to find out the reason. But if you want to have the best evaluation done, consult an otolaryngologist who is a specialist in throat, mouth and nose problems and their cures.

# Snoring By Nature Is...

Ever since a pioneer invented a device for curing snoring by attaching a sock with a tennis ball to the back of a shirt to prevent him/her from lying on the back, hundreds of other inventions have been made in the same field. These devices, sadly, initiate a very unpleasant stimulus every time you snore or do anything that can trigger snoring. Snoring is not a voluntary action. So if a device does keep you from snoring, it might also keep you awake all night.

Abnormality of the air passage is the root cause of snoring. When free flow of air which is required for normal breathing is hindered by some problem, it is highly likely that air strikes the back of the nose and mouth continuously. This vibration comes out as snoring.

Many people take snoring lightly imagining that it will not cause any harm. Contrary to this, people who suffer from snoring may in the long run, have serious health problems like obstructive sleep apnea. Apart from this, they cannot get a good night's rest and thus are deprived of complete rest. Also, it may embarrass the person and also disturb his/her spouse/bedmate.

Obstructive sleep apnea is a condition where snoring is interspersed with instants where the person completely stops breathing. These instances may occur for 10 seconds each unto 10 times each hour. Thus the sufferer may have 30 to 300 such episodes in a single night.

These reduce the oxygen levels in our blood and causes the heart to pump harder than normal.

A person is forced to sleep only lightly so that he can keep his muscles taut. Only this can regulate normal flow of air in a person's air pipe. This unrelaxed rest is not sufficient for the human body. This makes him less productive for the entire day and also lead to heart enlargement and heightened blood pressure

The following are some of the contributors to snoring:

**Anatomy of the mouth**

Tissues in the air passage are some of the factors of snoring. Narrowing of the air passage is itself a chief cause of snoring. Elongated soft palette, thickened soft palette, enlarged tonsils can all cause narrowing of this passage. All these cause obstruction of free air flow.

**Drinking just before bedtime:**

Most of the effective causes of snoring are those which make the throat muscles relax in excess. Alcohol being a sedative does just this. It acts as a relaxant on the throat muscles. Thus, consumption of alcohol just before sleeping can cause snoring.

**Apnea**

All too often, snoring and obstructive sleep apnea are found to be interrelated. So for any fitting treatment to be carried out, you must make sure that you are thoroughly diagnosed.

## Nasal problems

Various biological factors may also lead to poor air flow through the nose. The nasal bridge or septum as technically referred to is the underlying factor. When there is nasal congestion or when it is out of shape (crooked), there are greater chances of snoring.

There are many different methods to control and cure snoring, but one of the best permanent cures for snoring is surgery.

It is best to detect the cause of snoring very early since it will be easier to cure it. It is not fatal or even very damaging on health but more you procrastinate, the more severe the condition is likely to get.

## Snoring Help: Cures Against The Nocturnal Dilemma

An average human spends almost half his life sleeping. We achieve whatever we can in the remaining hours. Many people are successful at sleeping well, but there are some who don't and some just cant sleep peacefully.

Among these people, come the snorers. They are constantly woken up subconsciously because of the lack of sufficient amount of air and also due to snoring.

These people keep praying that they will get a good night's sleep. But when they finally realize that they can't, they turn to remedial measures for it.

If you are one of these, you can relax. There are many ways to cure it temporarily or permanently. The only thing you need to do is find these cures and be ready to face the minor risks that may be bundled with them.

The preliminary step is knowing why you snore. Once the cause is zeroed down on, the cure can be found. This is commonly seen in diseases whose immediate cause is not known. They don't have immediate cures. The ad-hoc cures help relieve the sufferer to a small extent and the rest is in the hands of fate.

A high percentage of people who are overweight snore. So shed your extra pounds as soon as possible. Because of accumulation of fat in their throat, they have narrower air passages increasing chances of vibration. Fleshier air passages also increase the chances of resonance of this sound.

Do not take relaxants just before sleeping. Overly relaxed muscles have a tendency to flip flap and this leads to blockage of the air passage. This is why we snore only while sleeping and not while we are awake. Our muscles like the rest of our body, relaxes when we sleep. People who snore are often advised to sleep lightly so that their muscles are kept tight.

Don't consume dairy products right before your bed time. These can lead to formation of mucus in the windpipe which further leads to snoring.

Sleep on your sides. Lying on your back is well known to aggravate snoring.

Sleeping at a regular time everyday makes your body adjust its body cycle likewise. So even if you do snore, you will get a good night's rest. The lost sleep due to snoring can be compensated by developing a good sleep schedule and thoroughly relaxing your body.

Make your pillows harder. This makes your throat muscles tighten. Since only over relaxed muscles lead to snoring. So hard pillows can help alleviate snoring.

Keep your throat wet at all times to lessen this congestion.

Smoking eats away your lungs in the long run. In a short while itself, however, it alters the cells of your throat to make them tougher to adapt to the harsh substances in smoke. This causes snoring. Swelling and inflammation of the respiratory tract also arise from smoking.

Nasal strips which help a person breathe comfortably by clearing the air pipe are found to be effective at controlling snoring. Some people find anti snoring sprays and pills to be of greatest effect.

Hundreds of snoring-control devices have been innovated ranging from nasal valve dilators to beds whose elevation you can adjust. These are available both online and offline.

Don't anticipate every product to work. They normally work since they were kept keeping the following specific need in mind - To cure you of your nightmare.

## Contributing Factors And Subsequent Snoring Remedies

Snoring is the annoying drumming noise that is produced by the throat along with its various components when they vibrate. It does not occur when you are awake. But when you are asleep, these tissues relax and blocks the normal passage for flow of air. This narrowing of the passage and inhibition of normal air flow causes snoring.

All remedial measures to snoring involve probing the cause of snoring. Only when the cause is known, can any concrete steps be taken to cure it. If not, one has to somehow find out the cause. The following can be the causes.

### 1. Obesity

Sedentary life, rich food, junk food and physiological problems cause people to develop all the conditions that could eventually lead to snoring. Obesity is one of these conditions. It is well known that people who are overweight snore more than those who have their muscles toned. The fleshiness of their throat is the chief cause of this. This there is more blockade in their throats. To counter this, the overweight people are often advised to relieve themselves of a few extra pounds. Shedding these extra pounds not alone alleviates them of snoring, but also improves their overall health.

## 2. Drinking

Do not consume alcohol just before sleeping. If you do, then your throat muscles will over relax and droop into the airway blocking it. This aggravates snoring.

## 3. Smoking

Smoking modifies the cells in the throat among all its other ill effects. The throat generates more mucus to withstand the passage of smoke and nicotine through the air tract so that there will be no inflammation. But the accumulation of mucus itself causes a blockade to air and hence snoring occurs.

## 4. Sleep pattern

There are stages of sleep. Stage1 sleep is when a person just begins sleeping. Every time a person is disturbed, he goes back to stage1 sleep. The second stage is Rapid Eye Movement (REM) sleep where dreams occur

Normally those who snore have a very irregular breathing pattern arising out of the grunts of their bed mates.

One should have good sleeping habits and practice sleeping at around the same time everyday to prevent snoring. Since a body requires 8 hours to rejuvenate, it is recommended that you establish a good sleep pattern.

## 5. Sleeping habits

People who sleep on their back snore more than those who sleep in other positions. This is because when you sleep on your back, gravity causes your tongue to withdraw to the back of your throat. Apart from this, the tissues in the throat dangle and this air that passes has to push these muscles up to pass. This causes them to vibrate and cause snoring.

It has been observed that sleeping in an elevated position reduces chances of snoring. At an angle of 30 degrees, the tongue wont roll back and the diaphragm will relax well.

## 6. Medical Problems

Peaceful sleep is lost when you have a blockage in the throat. This can be caused by inflammation that arises from allergies or infection. Tonsillitis, large adenoids, accumulation of excess mass in the throat and modification in cell contraction can block the flow of air in the throat. Surgery is commonly advised for snoring that arises of these complications

# Stop Snoring For Better Rest

It happens every night in homes all over the world. People retire to their beds after a long day filled with stress and excitement only to find more stress. The stress that afflicts many people during the night has to deal with a snoring spouse or partner.

Snoring accounts for many lost hours of sleep each night. The lost sleep is not just an issue for the men or women who are in the bed next to the snorer. Other family members can lose sleep over the problem as well. The booming sound of the snoring might reverberate throughout an entire house, with little escape for those left struggling to sleep against the noise.

For many people though, the issue of snoring reaches far beyond just the annoyance and frustration of the sound. For some people snoring is a symptom of a much more serious problem. That problem is sleep apnea, when a person who is asleep stops breathing. If you live with a snorer who sleeps deeply, you may have been witness to this without even realizing it. Often a person who is snoring falls into a rhythmic breathing pattern that is saturated with loud intakes of breath. As they breathe out they make a noise which is the snoring that other people hear. If that person ever seems to catch their breath, the snoring might stop momentarily, that silence could be the beginning of sleep apnea.

There are many remedies that claim to quiet the unruly noise that emanates from the snorer. Everything to adhesive strips that are said to open the nose passages to in serious cases, surgery to correct breathing problems. If the snoring is changing the sleep patterns of either the snorer or their family members trying a few approaches to halting the noise is a great idea.

It's even been suggested that snoring can be a symptom of something as simple as an allergy to either an environmental agent or even a particular food. The person might eat something for dinner and then later that evening, roll into a deep, noisy sleep. Monitoring the diet is a great first step to determine if the snoring occurs more frequently after a particular food is eaten.

There are also many natural supplements that are said to aid in helping to stop the problem of snoring. Some of them are directed at helping the snorer by relaxing the muscles that often are associated with the snoring. Others are geared towards addressing some of the other issues that have long been thought to contribute to snoring; things like being overweight or inactive.

How you sleep might also play a role in whether or not you are having a sleep that is peaceful for everyone around you. It's been suggested that if you sleep on your back you might be more prone to snoring. By adjusting the bed to encourage your body to remain on its side, the issue of snoring might become mute.

Researching new techniques and taking the time to investigate what works for you could mean a long and peaceful sleep for everyone involved. There are ways to stop snoring and once you find the solution your family will be eternally grateful.

# A Consistent Sleep Pattern Can Help Stop Snoring

During the week when you're working you might try and get to bed at a decent hour. You realize and recognize that a full eight or nine hours of sleep each night is essential to focus and productivity at work. When the weekend rolls around, you decide to go out and party and as a result you don't get to bed until the crack of dawn. The difference might not only be your bedtime or the hours of sleep you get but it might also be whether or not you snore.

Going to bed at the same time each night and sleeping the same amount of hours can have a direct impact on snoring. Snoring is never a good thing and it's sometimes a very sore spot in a relationship, especially when it's keeping one partner awake almost every night. The cause of the snoring could be contributed to a lack of sleep. Our bodies crave routine be it in the form of exercise, the number of calories we consume, and also how much sleep we are giving it every night.

Our bodies depend on sleep to remain rested and

vital. Routine is good and when our body is forced out of that routine, whether that be because of illness, stress or in this case a lack of sleep it can cause a person to snore. Snoring results in a fitful sleep that might leave the person feeling more tired than before they went to bed. It can also directly change the sleep patterns of those that the snorer lives with.

For someone who has a snoring problem, the idea of a scheduled pattern of sleep is well worth trying. It involves going to bed each night at approximately the same time and waking the next morning at a predetermined time. The use of an alarm clock is very helpful. Over time you might even notice that your body will develop its own inner clock and you'll awaken just before the alarm clock rings, after a nice free of snoring.

By developing this type of sleep pattern, the person will have less chance of snoring. Their body will be following a regular routine and that results in a feeling of being rested which is essential to good health.

Sound sleep is often a contributing factor in whether

or not a person snores. The difference between sleeping in a very quiet room as opposed to a room where there is outside noise filtering in can also playing a role in snoring.

If your goal is to stop snoring, it's important to establish a regular sleep routine and stick to it all week long. Your body will appreciate the regularity and with the added bonus of being rested, the chances of you snoring decrease. Pick a time to go to bed that you can live with and a time that's easy to wake up to each day. Stick to it and you may just stop your snoring.

# Losing Weight Can Help Stop Snoring

For anyone who has lived with a snorer they will tell you that the idea of having a restful night that isn't filled with the constant sound coming from their partner would be priceless. Many people see snoring as something of a win at the unlucky lottery. It fits into the "worse" category of the "for better or for worse" part of the marriage vows. However there may be a solution to that noisy problem that has another beneficial side effect as well.

Losing weight might be the answer to the snoring problem. When a person is overweight they will often also snore. By taking off some of the excess pounds the snoring will stop. The reason for this is because some people hold excess weight around their chests and neck areas. The added pressure weighs the muscles down and hence they snore. As they gain weight the snoring problem may worsen to the point that their spouse has to leave the room to sleep elsewhere. This can and often does ultimately affect the marriage or relationship. In cases like that, it's obvious that finding a way to stop the snoring is terribly important, and doing so before the problem reaches a point where the relationship is damaged should be the ultimate goal.

The difference between a quiet, restful sleep and a fitful, noisy sleep might not be more than a few pounds. One of the more effective ways to lose weight is to exercise. This serves a dual purpose since it is also believed that exercise has a positive effect on snoring too.

Eating a healthy diet is always a good idea. When we consume healthy foods in moderation our bodies will react by slimming down. Realizing that by accomplishing a weight loss goal you may also be ending the problem of snoring, can bump up your willpower a great deal.

Snoring can be the cause of a difficult sleep for not only the person living with the snorer but the person doing the snoring as well. Changing eating habits and getting out and exercising are natural and healthy ways to combat the snoring. By looking at the weight problem as a solution to the snoring problem it can be a strong factor in convincing a person that they truly are killing two birds with one diet, so to speak. Losing weight does not have to be about drastically restricting calories and exercising for hours each day. Instead it can be about consciously choosing what to eat each day, recognizing the value in a balanced diet and moving your body to not only shed some pounds but to strengthen it as well.

In the end you'll find yourself with not only a great looking outside but with a quieter inside. Snoring is a problem that can be stopped and wanting to do that for not only yourself but those who have to be subjected to the noise night-after-night is a great way to give the gift of silence.

# Natural Supplements Can
# Help Stop Snoring

For anyone who has spent even one night with a snorer, they will tell you that a solution to the problem is worth almost anything. Snoring is a chronic condition for many men and women and its effects are longer reaching than many people realize. Snoring accounts for many lost hours of sleep which translates into a loss of clarity and focus for some people. It's even been suggested that snoring is responsible for many hours of lost work.

The good news is that snoring is a condition that can be treated. The snoring can be stopped. One method that some people are turning to is the natural supplement solution.

There are products that have been introduced that claim to quiet the roaring boom of the snorer. Some of these products are all natural and are composed of substances taken straight from Mother Nature's bounty. For people who don't like the idea of turning to a prescription medication to stop their snoring, these natural supplements offer a perfect solution.

One such product that has been in the spotlight as of late is in the form of a spray. The spray is made from natural ingredients and the snorer simply points it towards the back of their throats before going to bed each night and it claims to act like a lubricant allowing the flow of air through the throat during the night. This type of product is appealing as a method of stopping snoring because in addition to be completely natural it's very simple to use. Also the fact that it is all natural is comforting for people who want to address the issue of their snoring without the added worry of using a prescription medication that might have adverse side effects.

Another natural remedy that may work to quiet the loud snoring sleeper is a tablet that contains herbs that work naturally at reducing the amount of mucous in a person's throat. Sometimes when a person is feeling congested, that congestion is coating some of the muscles in the throat which narrows the airway. If this happens one of the results can be that the person will snore.
They may not even be aware that the congestion is contributing to their snoring. By taking a natural

supplement that works at breaking up the mucous, they will find it easier to breathe both during the day and at night. This can have a significant effect on how loud they snore and in some cases it may quiet the snoring completely.

There are natural approaches to dealing with the problem of chronic snoring. Investigating the probable cause of the snoring and then researching the alternatives by either talking to an expert in natural medicine or visiting a health food store is a great first step to addressing the problem. It is reassuring to know that the way to stop your snoring might be a simple and natural remedy. Trying a natural remedy to cure your snoring problem can be both safe and effective.

# Exercise Can Help Stop Snoring

Snoring is a problem that affects numerous people all over the globe each night. It's so serious in some cases that it can ultimately lead to the end of a relationship. Sleep is a vital component in living a healthy and stress-free life and if your sleep is being disturbed by your own snoring or the snoring problem of a partner, it might be time to take some action.

There are numerous treatments available for those who snore including medication, tricks to keep you sleeping in a certain position or in extreme cases surgery. The solution to stop snoring might not be something that requires more than a few moments of physical activity each day. Exercise might be the answer to the snoring question.

One of the common causes of snoring seems to be excess body weight. Using exercise as part of a program to lose weight can also have the added benefit of stopping your snoring. This is by far the most natural way to quiet those nightly demons.

The exercise need not be strenuous. Even something as simple as walking each day can have an enormous impact on the person snoring. Their bodies become toned and at the same time the extra weight that they have been carrying around their throats melts away and over time the snoring quiets and eventually may disappear all together.

Swimming, hiking or riding a bicycle are all excellent methods of exercising the body. If done outside they add the extra benefit of getting the individual breathing fresh air and enjoying the elements. It can be refreshing for someone who often suffers from a fitful sleep because of snoring.

It's important to choose an activity that is appealing to you. It's also important to recognize that while exercising might not be your first choice of activity it can be vitally important to a healthy and balanced life particularly in the case of someone who snores. Snoring has many side effects including loss of sleep, loss of energy, less productivity at work and less motivation to do things. This can change a person's life; often in a very negative way.

For people who snore that are single, often the reason that they haven't pursued a committed relationship is because they are embarrassed by their snoring. This can lead to a sense of depression and self-doubt which in some people leads to the urge to overeat. They are jumping into a bitter cycle, gaining weight because they are eating to forget the snoring problem. Yet the increased eating leads to more weight which contributes to the snoring.

If you are married or partners with a snorer, it's beneficial to encourage them to exercise this is especially true if they are significantly overweight. People who are obese often suffer from a condition that can result in their breathing stopping while they are asleep. It is called sleep apnea and one of the symptoms of the condition is snoring. This is a serious medical condition and it can be treated by simply losing weight.

Stopping snoring by losing weight is a wonderful way to take care of not only your sleep problems but your entire body.

# Hypnotism Can Help Stop Snoring

If you have lived with a snorer for any length of time, you've probably tossed and turned through a few sleepless nights. Short of taping the snoring person's nose closed to quiet them or finding ear plugs that completely block the sound, you haven't been able to find a solution.

For some people the remedy to stop snoring might come in the form of hypnosis. For centuries people have been turning to hypnosis for many reasons. In recent years, one of those reasons is to stop snoring.

If you've ever watched a stage show that featured a hypnotist you might have witnessed people acting silly and taking on personas that weren't their own. The same idea behind that is used to address issues such as smoking, weight loss and even snoring. By relaxing and being hypnotized the person who is snoring can find the relief that they desperately seek.

Hypnotism involves tapping into the subconscious mind through a series of very specific techniques.  A trained hypnotist leads the person to a place where they feel utterly relaxed, than through the use of suggestions the person can literally change the way they think and feel. For some people this can be the solution to life-changing problems including snoring.

There are numerous audio recordings available that offer the chance to be hypnotized to stop snoring in the comfort of your own home. They generally come with instructions and they suggest that if followed correctly, snoring will soon be nothing more than a distant memory. For someone uncomfortable with the idea of visiting a hypnotist this might be a satisfactory solution. They simply listen to the recording and their mind will take over blocking the snoring. This approach doesn't work for everyone and an alternative might be to visit a hypnotist in person.

It's important to research a hypnotist before you decide to undergo hypnosis as a solution to help you stop snoring. Training is essential and it's also crucial to visit someone who has had success in working with people who have snored in the past. Hypnosis is not an area that everyone is familiar with so being certain that you are making an informed decision is essential to success. Choosing a professional with whom you feel comfortable and confident can be the foundation for a good experience. It's wonderful to imagine that your snoring can be stopped with the aid of someone who can reach into your mind and adjust the body so snoring doesn't occur anymore.

Not everyone can be hypnotized. Some people subconsciously resist it, but if you do find that you are able to relax to the point where you are open and receptive to the suggestions involved with quieting a snoring problem, than it can work for you. Many people have had success with using hypnotism to stop snoring. If snoring is having an impact on your life or the lives of those around you, than finding a trained and experienced hypnotist could be the first step to a lifetime free of snoring.

# Quitting Smoking Can Help
## Stop Snoring

If you smoke you've already been subjected to all the literature and information that details how damaging that habit can be to your health. You know about the impact of the chemicals in cigarettes on not only your lungs but your heart. Smoking can contribute to another problem that is wide-spread and creates conflict in many homes, that problem is snoring.

If a person smokes they are generally more likely to snore. The reasoning behind this is quite simple. The chemicals found in cigarettes and cigars cause changes in the tissue of the throat. When this tissue becomes irritated it can make a difference in how air flows through the throat. This difference is often what results in snoring. The air is obstructed in some way and it shifts, causing a change in how the person is breathing. The person affected might not even realize that their snoring is related to the fact that they smoke.

Snoring is a serious condition that can drastically

impact the lives of not only the person afflicted with it but those around them. Smoking is much the same. Its damaging effects are documented and if a person is smoking around others, those same consequences can affect them. The same can be said of snoring which changes the lives of others by stealing hours of sleep from them and by causing unnecessary stress and frustration.

Making a decision to stop smoking will have an impact on your health almost immediately. The person will generally feel more energized and will find it easier to breathe. It is that change that can directly influence whether or not they snore. With an air passage that is not clogged with the chemicals from cigarettes, the flow of air is smooth.

If the throat tissues aren't irritated than there is a likely chance that the person won't snore. This will result in them feeling more rested, more alert and having the ability to focus on things in a much clearer way. This can change a person's life significantly. If years have been spent struggling with the problem of snoring. Having that burden lifted from your life can drastically change everything from how you perform at your job to how fulfilling your marriage is. Quitting smoking can be a healthy and beneficial method of stopping a snoring problem.

Research has suggested that if a person stops smoking it might have an immediate impact on their snoring. Some people notice a change in their sleep patterns within days of having their last cigarette. This change can occur regardless of how long you have been smoking. If you are snoring as a result of smoking, whether you are a teenager experimenting with tobacco or a senior who has smoked their entire life, stopping now can also finally stop the snoring problem which may have been plaguing you for years. It's a positive step in a healthy direction and butting out can also silence the snores that have bothered you for years.

## The Connection Between Dairy Products And Snoring

When we or a person we love snores, we often try and do everything we can to remedy the problem. Stopping the snoring by discovering its cause can become a futile mission if we aren't looking in the right direction. If exercise, dieting, or natural health aids haven't won the snoring war it might be time to look in another direction. The answer to quieting the rumblings of a snorer might be in that glass of milk they had with their dinner.

Milk contains materials that can produce mucous in some people. There's an old wives tale that suggests that if you have a head cold you shouldn't drink milk. The reasoning is that the milk will contribute to the build-up of mucous that is already present and make the person suffering from the cold that much worse. Their nose becomes stuffier, their chest might feel congested and it becomes more difficult to breathe. It's that idea that leads some people to avoid the consumption of dairy products before bed. They believe that if they drink a glass of warm milk to help them fall asleep, that sleep with be riddled with the sounds of snoring. The milk producing mucous which becomes lodged within the throat passage and causes a narrowing which leaves less room for breathing, hence the resulting noise we refer to as snoring. If you are dining later and consuming milk it might be worth noting if you snore that night or if you snore when normally you don't. If you do discover that this is true, than the next step would obviously be to restrict your dairy intake or to consume products from the dairy family earlier in the day so your body has time to digest them before bedtime. If you rely on the milk you are drinking with your evening meal as a form of daily calcium, perhaps try drinking it with breakfast or lunch instead. Those few hours might make all the difference in whether or not you snore.

Adults aren't the only ones who snore. Often you can hear your infant or child while they sleep. Their breathing perhaps not as loud as your spouses when they are snoring, but it's evident that the subtle drone coming from your offspring is snoring in some form. The idea that milk and dairy products contribute to snoring is illustrated by the fact that children do snore. They consume, on average, more milk than most adults. For a child who tends to develop mucous build-up their breathing might be even more pronounced after they've had a dinner that included several servings of dairy products.

Although it's not wise to limit your child's intake of dairy if they are snoring, it could be a great and effective alternative for someone older. By choosing to take a calcium supplement as a replacement for a glass or two of milk, you could come out on the winning end by finding a peaceful night's sleep that's free of snoring.

# The Connection Between
# Alcohol And Snoring

It's relaxing and pleasurable to hit the bar after work with some friends. It gives you a chance to unwind and share a cocktail or two before you head home to bed. That stop at the bar might be costing you more than the price of a drink or two though. It might be costing you a night that doesn't involve waking up tired.

Alcohol can cause snoring. By partaking of a drink or two you can be setting yourself up to snore. The reason is that when we drink our bodies become relaxed, this includes the muscles of the throat. Often when a person has drank a few cocktails they will fall into a very deep sleep, a very relaxed sleep which can result in very loud snoring. If you've ever been at a party or social gathering where someone has consumed too much alcohol and fallen asleep, you might remember that they were snoring, and if you told them after, they'd say that they don't snore. That just might be true often a person only snores when they have been drinking liquor.

To stop the snoring they need to first become aware that their drinking is contributing to the seriousness of the problem. For someone in a relationship, their significant other will probably complain enough about the sound of the snoring and its effects that no other reminder will be necessary. For others, it might be that their snoring wakes themselves up. This can occur if the snoring is particularly loud and the person is sleeping restlessly. They'll find themselves jolted awake and wondering what was the cause. The cause is almost always that the snoring has startled them enough to wake them from their slumber. It's very hard to recognize this yourself though, after all how can we hear ourselves snore when we are asleep, especially a very deep sleep that results from the relaxing effects of alcohol.

The best and easiest way to remedy snoring that is caused by alcohol consumption is to either drink less or in some cases, not drink liquor at all. If this isn't an acceptable option another alternative might be to switch to another type of drink. Some beverages contain a higher concentration of alcohol than others. If you are snoring because you've been drinking a few glasses of wine, switching to beer might greatly improve the situation.

Another approach to stopping your snoring when it's brought on by drinking is to eat more while you consume the alcohol. Eating while drinking spirits can help you absorb less of the alcohol into your system. For someone who snores because of alcohol this can be very significant, it allows them to drink while at the same time, their sleep that night won't be too deeply affected by snoring.

If snoring is being brought on because of that beer that you drink with your dinner, it might be time to switch to a soda or a glass of water. Weighing the pleasure of the drink against the possibility of stopping snoring is a personal choice.

## Limiting Eating Before Bedtime Can Help Stop Snoring

It's getting to close to bedtime and your stomach is looking for a late night snack. You go to the kitchen and decide on a nice thick slice of chocolate cake. After brushing your teeth you tuck yourself into bed and within hours you feel the familiar hand of your spouse trying to wake you up so you'll stop snoring.

Snoring is a problem that almost everyone has had to deal with at some point. Whether it was a parent who snored, a partner or their own snoring problem, it changed not only their sleep patterns but their stress level as well. If we don't get a good night's rest we can end up irritated, frustrated and angry with the person who snores, even if logically it seems that there is nothing they can do about it.

There might be something that can easily change the situation and help them to stop snoring. The solution might be found in their menu. The foods we eat can have a direct impact on whether or not we snore.

Eating right before you retire for the night gives your body less of a chance to digest the food. This can result in the food sitting within your stomach and depending on the size of the snack or the meal it can also cause you to feel pressure on your diaphragm. It is that pressure that can result in snoring.

Adjusting your meal time might help improve the snoring. If you are accustomed to eating dinner later in the evening at eight or nine o'clock, it might be wise to move that ahead several hours so that by the time you do hit the hay, the food will have been digested and it won't result in a restless sleep that is filled with the sounds of snoring.

Experimenting a bit with eating times is wise in this case. It might be as simple as an hour difference in time that results in you snoring or not. That is a small change that can have a big result in not only your sleep but in the sleep of those who have listened to you snore night after night.

Snacks are often a regular routine of night time television viewing. Eating potato chips, popcorn or pretzels is a great way to add flavor to an evening of sports or movies. Choosing a different snack might help you to have a sounder sleep though. Some research suggests that honey has a positive effect on the airways and can help stop snoring. Eating an apple dipped in honey or having a cup of warm tea with honey will not only help with stopping the snoring but it won't place such a heavy burden on your digestive system at the end of the day.

Overall the main points to remember when eating to avoid snoring are:

- Avoid eating late in the day.
- Avoid eating snacks that contain too many calories
- Avoid snacks that take a long time to digest.

Looking carefully at your diet and your dietary habits might result in not only a healthier eating pattern but also may help with a snoring problem. Simply adjusting what you eat and when you eat it could stop your snoring completely.

# Bonus Chapter: Stress Relief

## About Stress Relief

The topic of stress relief has been the object of controversy in recent decades due to the various ways to administer it. There are different ways for different cultures. Where the Hindus have yoga the Japanese have Zen. Both of these methods are excellent in relieving stress. There are many types of yoga and this practice includes stretching of the muscles and various positions to relax each body part. Meditation and concentration for each movement will eventually with continued effort give you a youthful glow and allow you to keep stress levels at a minimum. Zen, on the other, hand is a style focusing on more of the meditation. Zen is a more philosophical approach to stress relief and really works if practiced on a regular schedule.

Other ways to relieve stress include deep breathing exercises, light physical exercise, reading, getting out into nature, the calming effects of light music; each individual has their own method. Some may prefer bingo or bowling while another may choose baking or smoking a cigarette.

Whatever the choice, there are certain consequences. For instance, if you choose to smoke to relieve your stress it may not be the best solution and could result in a health risk. Other ways to relieve stress are acupuncture and hypnosis. These must only be done by a professional. To locate a professional simply use the internet or it's as easy as your phone book under physicians or alternative medicine.

When you decide that relieving your stress level is what has to be done, consult your doctor. He or she will be able to determine whether your chosen method will be the best for you, and any adverse effects will then be discussed. Your physician may prescribe medication for you if you are at a risk for other problems. The problem about stress relief is to not do anything at all. Some people are not aware they are at risk for problems such as heart attack and stroke.

**Anxiety Symptoms Relief Disorder: When Cures Are Not Working**

There are many people in this world who are in the clutches of anxiety and they seek help from various sources in order to get away from these even taking extreme measures like ignoring its debilitating effects. There are many people who have reduced the suffering of anxiety through these sources but at the same time there are many people who suffer more from its treatments. This state is called 'Anxiety Symptoms Relief Disorder'.

Actually there is no term called 'Anxiety Symptoms Relief Disorder' it is basically an attempt made in order to cure a person's anxiety but the end result is failure. We cannot say that the cause of this failed attempt is a disorder. It is used basically to describe the state of mind of some people when they are not cured from Anxiety. For instance those people who are forced to face the treatment by family members may believe that there is nobody to help them in that state or when they create a false belief that their disease cannot be cured, such people are basically prone to Anxiety Symptoms Relief Disorder. This is basically a psychological problem where the person who is facing this is taken care of first and then comes the treatment of his\her anxiety along with their other problems.

The term 'Anxiety Symptoms Relief Disorder' does not show up as a recognized medical term in any book so we can say that this term is not exactly a recognized medical phrase. There are many people around us who are undergoing this disorder for many years but when it comes to dealing of anxiety disorders there are many people who ignore the treatments that are available to them. This is a situation where the people suffering from anxiety may not easily accept the required diagnosis and there by the cures that are offered to them. This is a tough situation where anxiety disorder can take a person to a deep state of depression and there by lead them to suicidal thoughts.

The coining of the phrase 'Anxiety Symptoms Relief Disorder' is to make all understand that there are many people who go through this anxiety disorder and thereby creates a feeling within them that basically hinders the curing of anxiety related problems.

This is the situation where all those who suffer from anxiety disorder needs a lot of support from their family and friends. They should be provided with all the care and help from others and there by make them feel that they are not alone and this would help in an enormous way to tackle this and any other problems that may come in the way.

## Stress And Dreams

Nightmares are often seen by people under a lot of stress. Although it is not very clear whether stress is the reason for people to see nightmares or nightmares are one of the reasons for people to feel stress, but it is very clear that stress and dreams are interrelated.

Dreams are basically a part of the human subconscious, so there is enough possibility that these dreams act as the subconscious part of a person which helps him understand what is happening in him. Many people do not accept the fact that they are affected by stress disorders but in turn their mind denies this fact by making them dream about the same thoughts that bothers them.

They are many findings which show that stress causes nightmares. But this completely depends upon a person's mind fluctuations. People who are prone to stress disorder may often try to find out the source of their stress in their dreams, but some see dreams that helps them to get along with this disorder without any further complications. But apart from all this, there are other people who dream about stress which end up in horrifying nightmares. That is why people think that stress and dreams are connected.

In order to find out whether stress and dreams are inter connected a group students conducted a test about a subject for which they where going to have an exam in a few days. For this, the students were divided into two groups. Information was passed on to the first group that they will have a difficult exam. But for the second group no information was given. The result of this test was, the first group to whom the information about the difficult exam was passed had undergone stress by thinking about the difficulty they have to face all through the exam thereby making them dream about their failure in the exam which in turn gave them a few restless nights. Where as the second group to whom no information was given, did not show any symptoms of stress. The end result of this test was that the stress symptoms stopped the students from seeing positive dreams of exam and made them see the worry some exam which they have to face.

The test which was done for stress and dreams connection can also be a little inconclusive. The stress what the students faced may be due to some other case which was accompanied by the problematic situation. But in both ways it ends up in same conclusion that stress and dreams are interconnected as the stress factor stops a person from seeing positive dreams.

The Inter relation of stress and dreams was always a fascinating topic for all researchers. This is so because all studies and tests they have conducted till now have not shown any solid proof for the fact that stress symptoms make a person see nightmares and stops them from enjoying a beautiful dream.

## Using Music Therapy For Stress Relief

When it comes to your overall mental health, stress is the biggest problem that most of face. It is also the biggest reason for many health problems that we face daily. Most of don't even understand that stress can be the major cause of major health problems like heart problems.
There are many different types of therapy that can be used to help with stress relief and music therapy is a relaxing and soothing one that can help with stress but also major and minor illnesses as well.

Music therapy services are available to adults and children with disabilities. Sessions are individually designed according to each person's special needs.

Using music and music activities, the music therapist works with each individual to address specific goals and objectives that are determined by the therapist.

With music therapy both individual and small group sessions will be conducted with regular progress evaluations. Music therapy can be done for clients with the following disabilities: Autism, Cerebral Palsy, Down Syndrome, Mental Retardation, Attention Deficit Disorder, Lowe's Syndrome, and, Tourrette's Syndrome.

Music Therapy may be commonly defined as the structured use of music and music activities geared toward helping individuals with disabilities meet both musical and non-musical goals. Music therapy goals may be based on behavioral, physical, cognitive, social, and emotional or language and communication. Music is a proven relaxation technique as well as a stimulant. Those who use music therapy often experience positive changes.

Music therapy is good for people of all ages may benefit from music therapy, from young children to elderly seniors. People with almost any disability have ability when it comes to music. Music Therapy clients participate through playing instruments, improvising and making up new songs, singing, or even just listening. The people that are involved in Music Therapy sessions may range from having a mild learning disability to having severe mental retardation.

Music therapists assess clients' communication skills, social functioning, physical health and mobility, cognitive skills, and emotional well-being by how they respond to music. They design Music Therapy sessions for individuals according to their unique needs. In these tailored sessions, therapists use techniques such as music improvisation, receptive music listening, music performance on instruments and with the voice, and learning through music. That is just too cool. When you think of music in terms of therapy, it is very easy to forget how truly useful music can be. It really does sooth the savage beast within us if we let it.

**Using Art Therapy For Stress Relief**

One of the more fascinating measures taken for stress relief can be had with an art therapy. With so many different forms of therapy today it's tough to know which are the most effective for which condition, but art therapy enjoys great success in helping people suffering from a collection of conditions that are both physical and mental. If you are looking for an exciting method for relieving stress, art therapy is a good option.

An art therapy session will help you show others how art can lead to self awareness and understanding, as well as how soothing it can be to engage in the creative process. Taking the time to focus on a piece of art alone can make a tremendous difference in how we live and think and can reduce stress amazingly. Art therapy also helps people to discover things about themselves based on what they draw. It is a good tool that psychologists use in assessing their patients.

Receiving art therapy can be done at your own pace if you go about finding places that offer it online. This is great for those who have families and can't change their lives. Art therapy will help you to get a better understanding of yourself and your lifestyle. It is a great way for you to find and get rid of the problems that you may be facing. Many hospitals and doctors offices would recommend art therapy but it can be difficult to find the right place for you so be sure to do your research before signing up with anyone in particular.

If you can imagine all of the artists out there who use their art as a means of expressing themselves, it will be easier for you to see that you can do it too. You don't necessarily have to be a perfect artist to benefit from this type of therapy; however, it helps to use this therapy as a means of expressing yourself. It is a great resource for getting out those feelings which can often be harmful when not expressed. Art has always been used as a way to express oneself so why not make it a part of your stress relief regimen?

If you are having a hard time dealing with your everyday stresses and if you are wondering what you can do to help ease your stresses, you should consider art therapy as a means of helping you. It can't hurt to give it a try. With alternative medicine becoming a preferred way to dealing with life's problems, art therapy is just a drug free method of controlling your stress which can also help to reduce many of your common illnesses. Search online for art therapy classes in your area.

**Stress Relief Vacations**

Perhaps the most common and simplest form of reducing stress is to take a vacation. Nothing can work better for dealing with stress than to remove yourself completely form the source of it all together. Planning a vacation is the simplest way to do this. If you are trying to decide where you would like to go for your next vacation, you might want to consider an island resort. It can be a difficult choice with so many beautiful and exotic places to go to these days. For example if you've always wanted to go to the Caribbean or even Brazil. That's still a very large choice because there are so many resorts to visit in both of them.

If you decide to go to the Caribbean for example, you could choose to go to Jamaica, the Bahamas, or the island of Puerto Rico. There are also other very exotic possibilities like Antigua, Barbados, and St Lucia. That is not even the half of it. There are so many islands in the Caribbean that you could go to for that tropical honeymoon or anniversary celebration that choosing the best one can be nearly impossible.

Many people decide to buy an all inclusive resort packages because they make your island vacation much cheaper. One particular hot spot island that you can visit is Fiji. There are many all inclusive island resorts that you can choose from and the locations are often known for its great nightlife, especially during spring break. The long white sand beach is simply beautiful too.

The best part of an all inclusive island vacation is that everything that comes in your package for your nightly rate. You end up saving a lot of money in the long run going all inclusive and you don't have to worry about a thing on your vacation. Gourmet meals, drinks, snacks, water sports, lands ports, spa facilities, and fitness facilities are all included in one easy package so that you can just enjoy your vacation.

If you are currently planning an island resort vacation, you should visit your nearest travel agent and book an all inclusive package right away. That is the best way to ensure that you get your money's worth. Travel agents are partnered up with many hotels etc. so that you can save as much money as possible during your vacation. It certainly saves you a lot of money on souvenirs and other things too so that you can share your good times with those you love.

Dealing with stress is a lot better when you go to a great resort for relaxation. Most resorts offer you massage deals and packages as well as spa treatments etc. these are excellent for men and women and are often a part of the resort package. A foreign land to do it in simply adds icing to the cake. Why not take an excellent vacation for reducing your stress levels? It can be the best way to help you get your life in order and to get that much needed time to just sort things out and change your attitude all together.

## Have A Healthy Body And Mind For Stress Relief

When most of us think about our bodies and dealing with stress it is mostly just in terms of losing weight. Our weight is what we use to define our bodies these days. Food is the key to boosting your self esteem as well as reducing stress. Food should be taken in its natural form. When I say natural forms I mean for example, when you eat vegetable and fruit it helps to eat them in the form that they naturally come in. if you eat fruit from a can, it is contained in syrup and sugars that will not be good for you so eating them raw is the best choice.

When you are eating vegetables it is best to eat them raw and steamed because it keeps all of the vitamins and minerals in them. You should also avoid processed foods and fried meats.

Don't get me wrong fats are a necessary aspect of nutrition however saturated fats are not. The right balance of foods in a day can really be a key factor in reducing your stress levels as most fruits and vegetables contain mood enhancers that most of us don't even think of.

It is best to eat at least three meals a day that are balanced with each food group as prescribed by the food guide pyramid and in between snacks as well. What people don't know is that it is ideal that you eat five small meals a day instead in order to get the most our of your metabolic system. The more foods that you intake in a day that are healthy the better to boost your metabolism.

It is not always easy for most of us to follow the food guide pyramid; however, it is still the best way to ensure that you get the most out of your efforts. Diet and exercise combined is the best way too keep your stress levels at bay, but if you can't do both walking and eating right is the way to go. There is no real excuse not to do both, but it was necessary to mention them.

When we think of stress, we rarely think that food plays a part in it. The truth is that a balanced diet is your best tool in dealing with stress. Junk food and fast foods can actually become a depressant for most people. Foods that are high in fat can greatly reduce our moods. We often feel sluggish and tired after eating junk food. The right diet that is balanced can really have a good effect on your system and that includes your stress levels.

## Exercise Can Reduce Stress

Stress is not something that any of us enjoy going through, however, we are all forced to deal with the effects of stress sooner or later. When most of us think of stress we just assume that it is a fact of life that there is no cure for. That is not true. A healthy and balanced diet can reduce the effects that our bodies experience when under stress. However, regular exercise can also help with that as well.

When most of us think of adding exercise to our daily routines it is usually because of weight issues that we have. What is not so commonly known is how exercise can actually reduce stress and our body's reaction to it. It may sound silly but it is really true. The reason for it is because of the amount of energy we use in exercising. Every time we exercise we actually drain stress right out of our body all together. Think about it, if you went jogging and began in a stressed out mood or high strung, chances are that at the end of your jog, you are suddenly relaxed and feeling fine.

You don't have to go overboard on exercise in order to feel the effects of it either. In fact a walk in the morning will do a lot to help reduce your stress levels, and an added benefit to it is that you will also upgrade your fitness levels while loosing weight. If you take out even just a half of an hour during the day to exercise, you will notice that you sleep better at night, which will lessen your groggy and sleepy feelings during the day.

This will also help you in living a stress free lifestyle. It is a well known and documented fact that eating right and exercising regularly is great for maintaining a stress free life but it can't do everything on its own. You must also make time to be alone without any people around you to do things that interest you. Perhaps the best exercise you can take daily is walking or jogging. Even riding a bike can be a great way to reduce your stress. For example walking or riding a bike to work in good weather rather than driving. It gives your journey a purpose, which will make it easier to follow through with it.

Exercise alone cannot reduce your stress, but it can certainly help. A proper diet will also be a key to maintaining your stress levels. If your body is physically healthy, your ability handle stress is greatly increased. It is just a simple fact. If you are serious about keeping your stress under control, be sure to add exercise to your daily routine.

## Stress Affects Your Mental Health

Mental health issues that are caused by stress can range from homicidal or other violent acts towards oneself or drive others to addictions. The range of mental health disorders that are stress related is so broad that it can be difficult to understand how two situations fall in the same category. The days of shock therapy are gone for the most part, but it still is used for certain mental illnesses. Gone, too, is the routine procedure of frontal lobotomies to calm patients into total submissiveness.

A large key to dealing with stress related mental health issues is to know how to relieve stress. We now understand that men who are returning from wars endure thoughts and images that affect them in ways that we have only begun to be aware of. Post traumatic stress disorder which is caused by stress can affect victims of abuse and violence of all types. Only recently have we begun to understand how traumatic events can affect the people who survive them.

Despite the many types of mental health disorders that currently exist because of stress, some of them tend to be much more common than others. Mental health disorders are not discriminatory and affect everyone. They do not choose specific people or races to affect. Mental health disorders are equal opportunity problems. These disorders have been proven to be hereditary in some cases but that is the closest generalization that you can expect.

A very common mental illness that is caused by stress is manic/chronic depressive disorder. This is characterized by extreme highs and lows in moods for no apparent reason. Sufferers are irrational and quick to change, in terms of mood. For example, if you suffer from this disorder you are happy—very happy or sad--- very sad for no apparent reason. Stress is a major cause of this problem.

Eating disorders, which are also quite common, include anorexia (not eating), and bulimia (binging and purging) are also caused by stress that arises from self esteem. Anxiety disorders are characterized by having an irrational dread of living one's life, to the point where it is incapacitating.

Obsessive-compulsive disorder (OCD) is a form of anxiety disorder where a person obsesses (thinks about) and is compulsive (does) about a particular action such as washing their hands, to the point where he or she repeats this action an inordinate amount of times. Stress is a major aspect of our lives and can lead to serious mental problems if not taken under control. Learning to contain stress can lead to your overall health.

**Relieving Stress Through Stress-Management Websites**

A lot of Internet-uses consider it to be a boon not only because it is a vast reservoir of information, but also because it is a great reliever of stress. No individual is free from stress; everybody has to face it in one form or the other. The Internet offers a number of stress-management websites where people can obtain a certain degree of relief from the stress they face in life.

For instance, a stress-management website, such as Stress Less, teaches innovative methods of managing stress. On Stress Less, you can contact qualified professionals on the subject of stress, communicate with them privately, and obtain solutions to your stress-related problems.

Besides offering professional help in dealing with stress, several stress-management websites organize online anxiety- and stress-management programs that will help individuals deal with stress in an effective manner. These programs usually comprise modules that provide information on the fundamental cognitive behavioral techniques of stress management, reduction, and elimination. If you follow the tips and techniques that these stress-management websites offer, the quality of your life will improve, and you will develop a sense of peace and well-being.

Stress-management websites also teach users how to deal with stress with the help of techniques such as relaxation, deep breathing, progressive muscle relaxation, and meditation. You can purchase and download information on stress-management techniques at one of these stress-management websites. In addition, they comprise facilities such as tracking diaries, quizzes, inspirational emails, and many more not only to encourage you and provide you with the necessary inspiration to live life productively and fully, but also to help you get rid of the stress in your life.

You can gain relief from stress by making use of the instructions available at stress- management websites. Stress is usually the result of wrong thought patterns. These sites, therefore, teach you to develop a positive outlook on life.

Stress-management websites also use music as a major stress-relieving factor. You can get rid of a great deal of stress simply by listening to music. However, listening to any type of music won't relieve you of stress. You have to listen to a genre that you truly love and enjoy. Listening to sentimental music can help some people relax. Others can relax only if they listen to classical and instrumental music. Discover the genre that can help you relax and listen to it on a regular basis. This can help you get rid of stress.

The Internet offers myriad ways of getting rid of stress, and the sheer variety of it could confuse you a great deal. Ultimately, you have research the various methods and find out which stress- management website works best for you.

**Impacts Of Stress On The Mind And Body**

The impacts of stress on your mind and body are several. They could be categorized into emotional, mental, and physical impacts. The effects that stress has on the psychological conditions of an individual include behavioral and mental symptoms of stress. The emotional impacts of stress are those that are related to emotions or relationships.

People suffer a number of inconveniences due to the impacts of stress on their mind and body. The worst symptoms of stress are the physical symptoms, which include a rise in heart rate, muscular tension, backaches, chest pain, sleep disorders, nausea, frequent colds, and headaches. These symptoms might appear to be minor; however, if they are neglected, they could also lead to death.

The impacts of stress on a person's mind or behavior patterns can be dangerous unless they are taken care of immediately. In addition, the impacts of stress on a person's mind can also cause physical symptoms. The mental symptoms of stress include anxiety, loss of memory, poor judgment, indecisiveness, and loss of objectivity. Due to these symptoms, people under stress could develop eating disorders and eat lesser or more than they require. This could, in turn, result in obesity, high blood pressure, and ulcers. The impacts of stress on a person's mind can also lead to drug abuse or alcoholism, which could be the result of poor objectivity or lack of judgment.

The impacts of stress on a person's emotions could also lead to physical symptoms. For example, symptoms such as moodiness, loneliness, depression, irritability, restlessness can lead to several health disorders. Nervous and agitated people stand a greater risk of developing ulcers because their agitated condition gives rise to enhanced acid activity in their bodies. People who cannot relax due to stress and are, therefore, excessively restless also suffer from headaches that result from the constant stimulation to their brains caused by restlessness.
Depression can drive people to suicide or at least force them to attempt suicide.

If you don't take the required steps to manage stress properly, these symptoms or a mixture of some of these symptoms of stress can cause great harm to you.

**Stress Management Tips**

Tension is very familiar and something which most people cope with day by day. People frequently feel tension in sites that concern them, like acquiring a divorce, concern about losing their work, or worry over a kinsfolk being sick or undergoing a surgery.

Worry and stress go well together.

Day-after-day, people generally experience some sort of tension, which has both over emotional and forceful effects, producing either an affirmative or an antagonistic reaction. Although there's no such matter like a stress-free life, all people should find ways to aid them cope with tension, which fixes life gentler in the long run. Acquiring some tension management ways include working on changing your mindset so rather than worrying about such things you've no hold over, like losing your job, practice something affirmative such as sitting and doing up a job hunt . Besides panicking and worrying over things you can't change, tension management aids you read to solve problems.

Tension management may help all to learn to cope with

pessimistic tension in their own lives. Affirmative stress is really beneficial and includes results that make you concentrate, such as having an exam. Though nobody savors this, positive tension is what which makes a person study, and learns. Negative or prolonged tension is destructive and may cause physiological, psychical, and emotion troubles. Studies have associated antagonistic stress to hypertension, cardiopathy, depression, and many such problems.

People who don't use stress management frequently address self-medication like, alcohol, overeating, drugs, fits of uncontrollable anger, excessive sleeping, and other such things, which makes things even worse. Tension management aids people find fit ways to contract chronic stress like living a better lifestyle and finding affirmative ways to deal with problems.

Tension management makes you to focus on the affirmative, important affairs in your lifespan and not to concern about things you've absolutely no ascendance over. Rather than sitting and worrying, practice something physical like going for a nice walk, which would release endorphins and will make you feel good, aids in keeping you fit, and discards away stress. Do learn something new which will help you to relax like yoga or meditation. Also, Join a yoga union which meets 2 or 3 times per week so you will not only learn yoga but see fresh people and bask the cultural interaction. Tension management involves memorizing to forgive yourself of some of the errors you've made, spoiling yourself disregarding how engaged your life becomes, and having a affirmative outlook even while matters are not even liked by you.

**Stress Management Tips Help You Cope Better**

People all over the world will, at a time in their lives, cope with tension either in their own life or in the job. In today's high society, tension has become a common trouble and rather than reaching for medicine, there are a lot of tension management tips that aid persons cope with this. Although it's impossible to dispatch tension from your every day life, it's imaginable to acquire to boil down tension or deal with it utilizing tension management tips. The 1st of many tension management tips you would need to infer what is inducing the tension in your own life and overpowering you. Each day, people call their physicians as they feel disabled by their high tension levels, which would actually head to physical troubles and sickness. It's not merely people in the manpower searching help but other people like care givers looking after family members, individual parents, and couples who are trying to balance a family, responsibilities and work. Here are numerous tension management tips to aid people abiding from stress and their related problems.

Don't make your work the centre of your life but rather, find a fit balance between your work, your family, entertainment, responsibilities and things which you enjoy. People blank out how to enjoy life and relax, which makes them more inclined to depression, anxiousness disorders, tension, and other troubles. Taking a holiday without any cell or laptop is fantastic but in middle of the holidays, you should find something you enjoy doing and so make an aggressive effort to do so, specially during nerve-wracking times.

You deserve to relish yourself and should have fun, which many people appear to blank out. If you relish golfing, parks, museums, knitting, playing cards, jogging or taking walks on the country side, make a calculated attempt to admit these in your life. Employ biofeedback or speculation to lower your tension level and have mental relaxation. Brush off antagonistic thoughts and focus on only the affirmative things in life.

Tension management tips aid people infer that they don't have to experience guilty spending an relaxing day when your doing nothing. It's all right to turn off the pager, cell, or computer and take a break from everything. Whether you barely sit quietly and learn, get foul in garden, take a good bubble bath, also play with puppy, or see a movie with your family, just blanking out about your own problems awhile affords you altogether afresh outlook.

If tension management tips aren't aiding, particularly if you've no idea of what's inducing you to experience depression or stress, you should seek a master's help.

## Mental Stress - Indications And Relaxation Techniques

Problems people feel with tension are frequently shared into physical and the psychological. Mental tension symptoms that people might feel as they're abiding from excessive tension might include indications that strike both the conduct and the cognitive regions of their brain. A few of the mental tension indications that's affiliated with the cognitive region of an individual includes troubles with memory holding, lack of appropriate judgment, constant negativism, being a fusspot, irresolution and even uneasy thoughts. The mental tension indications that cope with an individual's conduct include neural tics or practices like frantic pacing or nail biting, short temper that might end in picking by battles and making apologies for not requiring accomplishing duties.

Mental tension indications sometimes can cause physical stress indications.

Lessons of such physical indications that root from these psychological stress indications include headaches, ulcers, weight gain or, migraines or even loss in weight. These physical indications might end from mental tension indications because of domino set up. If you're to analyze why an individual might acquire weight or reduce when strained, it is frequently due to the modified thinking that food may provide ease or that food isn't attracting. These are part of the tilt mental strain symptoms, deficiency of appropriate judgment or the departure of an individual's objectiveness.

However an individual can ease the troubles that stress may lay on his / her brain is something which can be chose from a couple of possibilities. The usage of easiness techniques to aid relieve stress besides as the mental strain indications and the physical strain symptoms which advance with it's gaining popularity. A relaxation method that people utilize while dealing with strain is yoga. A different possible strain reliever which uses relaxing as its significant agent is meditation. These 2 frequently come together and possibly used in alignment with the, or as replacement relaxation technique.

A different kind of relaxation that aids facilitate an individual from the effects which mental stress indications may add is Tai-Chi. This old Chinese military art accepts the fluid motions of the dissimilar Tai-Chi postures and utilizes these to produce the affirmative energy that accompanies the moves to help comfort the dismissive effects of tension.
Using some of the relaxation techniques given above and also other stress busting remedies will act as a welcome lifestyle change, sleeping habits and also the things which you eat might help ease an individual of the adverse issues of the psychological tension symptoms and physical tension symptoms.

**Exercise & Stress Relief- A Healthy Relationship**

In today's modern and fast life style a person can easily fall into the deep abyss of stress. There is no time for them to look over their needs after their work and managing their home and family. As time passes by we may never realize we are suffering from stress.

It's true that exercise to a great extent reduces stress. Doing exercise is not always enjoyable, but in this fast pace modern world it is a must in our daily lives. Take the case of cardiovascular exercise which moderates your emotions as they release endorphins during the exercise which acts as a natural pain reliever and boosts your mood. Due to this increase in endorphins, the exercise will reduce the stress from your body. This is why it is said that exercise and stress relief is related. During this process you will sweat it out which makes you feel relaxed, refreshed and get good a nights sleep.

Regular exercise usually keeps the body fit and mind stress free. In this busy world people always complain that they have no time for exercise, it is just a lame excuse they make as they find it's not enjoyable. But when you understand how closely exercise and stress relief is linked, you will automatically find out at least some time to do any some form of exercise.

Exercise need not always be a serious activity which requires you to sweat and pant. If you are a first timer to this, or have not exercised for a long while, you can just start slowly by doing some simple exercises.

You can also go for an activity that needs only very little preparation which can include gardening, taking your pet out for walk or cleaning up your house. By doing this you can make the transition easier and enjoyable.

If you are not in a good mood and if you don't feel like doing exercise give yourself a break before you go for a bigger more strenuous exercise. Then you can opt for ordinary activities like doing laundry, walking around the garden etc. Still if you do not want to do things on your own, you can ask support from your friend to come with you or attend a fitness program.

By doing exercise you will find all your problems seem less heavy. Playing your favorite sports along with your friends and enjoying your life in general, all these will reduce the effect of stress.

Some basic\important ideas on exercise and stress

relief:

- Exercise reduces your built up tensions and emotional tensions.
- Exercise release endorphins and other hormones giving the feeling of well being within you.
- Exercise can also be used as a means of social gathering and thereby building up a better social life.

To conclude, exercise calms your stress level and your nerves by making you feel much better about yourself. It provides a great opportunity to meet people and thereby maintaining a healthy relationship.

CPSIA information can be obtained
at www.ICGtesting.com
Printed in the USA
BVHW041441141220
595677BV00007B/190